Latrina Walden™
Exam Solutions

A Quick Reference Guide

Top Primary Care Medications and Disease Processes

www.latrinawaldenexamsolutions.com

Disclaimer

Legal Stuff – copyright 2023

Legal stuff

Products produced, published or sold by www.latrinawaldenexamsolutions.com including but not limited to blogs, podcasts, courses, digital materials and all other products are for entertainment and informational purposes only and should not be used to make medical diagnosis, give medical advice or prescribe medical treatment.

More legal stuff

These productions are designed to provide accurate information in regard to the subject matter covered and uses reasonable efforts to ensure that such information is accurate. LWES assumes no responsibility for correctness, accuracy or recommendations in the products or errors omissions or any outcomes related to your use of the products.

Mandatory legal stuff

LWES products may provide information, guidance and recommendations related to a variety of subject matters, including but not limited to, medical treatment, emergency care, drugs, medical devices and side effects; however research, clinical practice and government regulations often change the accepted standards and is solely your responsibility and not the responsibility of LWES to determine appropriate medical treatment, the use of any drug in the clinical setting, and for determining FDA status of a drug, reading the package insert and reviewing prescribing information for the most up to date recommendations on doe, precautions, and contraindication and determining the appropriate usage for a product.

Disclaimer

More legal mandatory stuff

Products are intended solely as a guide and for educational purposes are not intended to be used for actual medical treatment or as a statement of any standard of care. These products are provided as is and is available without warranty whether expressed or implied. You understand that your use of this is at your sole risk.

ISBN 978-1-7369010-6-9

9 781736 901069

How to Use This Book

ONLINE COURSE

There is an accompanying online course to this manual. You do not need it, but it is recommended. This is specifically for those who have visual needs in learning. The online course is separate and can be located at www.latrinawaldenexamsolutions.com

If you need help in locating the course contact us and our representative can assist you! Happy studying!

WHAT IS THIS COURSE?

This quick-reference book is your essential guide to the top disease processes and medications you'll encounter during your first one to two years in primary care and urgent care settings. Designed for fast-paced practice, it helps you swiftly find answers to pressing clinical questions, enabling you to provide comprehensive, holistic care to your patients. With a focus on efficiency, this resource equips you to navigate common challenges confidently, ensuring that you can deliver the best possible patient care without getting bogged down. Perfect for new practitioners, this book streamlines your workflow while keeping patient well-being at the forefront

WHO IS THIS FOR?

This quick-reference book covers the top medications and common disease processes you'll encounter in the first 2-3 years of working in primary care. Whether you're a Family Nurse Practitioner (FNP), Physician Assistant (PA), or MD, this resource is designed to guide your decision-making and improve patient care in primary care or urgent care settings. Perfect for quick consultations, it provides essential information to help you confidently manage your patients from day one.

How to Use This Book

WHY ARE SOME OF THE WORDS HIGHLIGHTED GREEN?

I've done this so we can specifically highlight the likely term you are going to see on your AANP or ANCC board exam.

WHY DON'T YOU DISCUSS THE ANTIBIOTICS IN DEPTH?

Because this is NOT how your boards are designed. Your boards do not arbitrarily discuss medications, let alone antibiotics randomly. When medications are an answer option, it is always in relationship to a treatment of a diagnosis or a side effect/contraindication. NEVER EVER has medication been tested on the exam in this manner. Trust me. If you are able to match the disease process with the corresponding 1st line treatment, then you are well on your way to passing your board exam.

This book is designed to be used while you are in school and when you are preparing to study for your AANP and ANCC board exam.

Table of Contents

RESPIRATORY

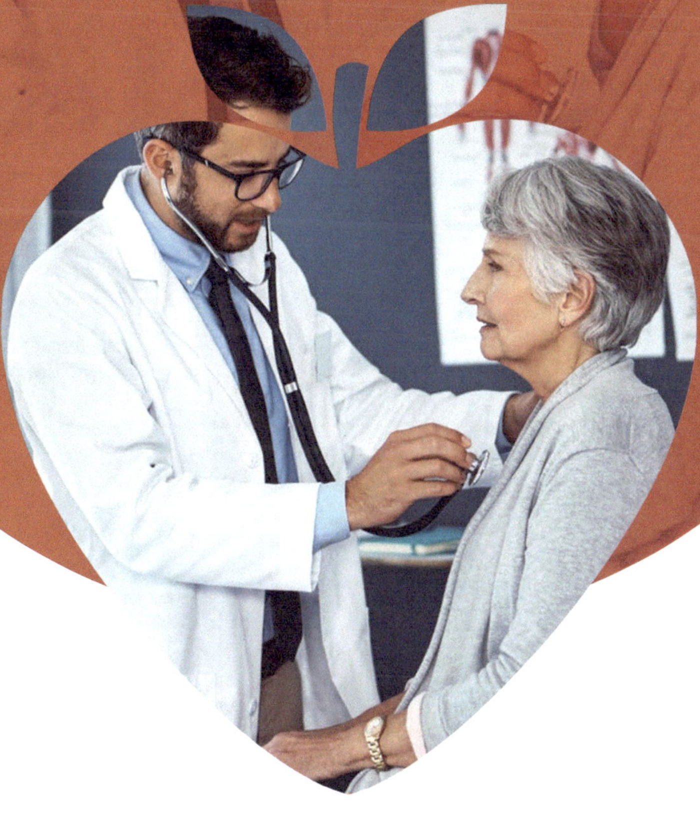

Latrina Walden™
Exam Solutions

RESPIRATORY

Citalopram

Definition of the disease

Asthma is a chronic respiratory condition characterized by inflammation of the airways, Bronchoconstriction (narrowing of the airways), and increased sensitivity of the airways to various stimuli. This chronic inflammation and Bronchoconstriction lead to recurrent episodes of wheezing, breathlessness, chest tightness, and coughing, especially at night or in the early morning. Asthma is a chronic condition that requires long-term management. Treatment typically involves the use of medications, including bronchodilators (such as short-acting or long-acting beta-agonists) to relieve symptoms and anti-inflammatory drugs (such as inhaled corticosteroids) to control inflammation and prevent exacerbations. Asthma management also includes identifying and avoiding triggers, monitoring symptoms, and having an action plan for dealing with acute episodes.

Brand Name	Generic Name	Classification
Ventolin, ProAir, AccuNeb, Vospire, Salbutamol, Proventil	**Albuterol**	**Short-Acting Beta-Agonist (SABA)**
Serevent, Fordil, Perforomist, Arcapta Neohaler	Salmeterol, Formoterol Indacaterol	Long acting beta agonist **(LABA)**
Flovent, Flonase, Pulmicort,Rhinocort, Asmanex	Fluticasone, Budesonide, Mometasone, Beclomethasone, Flunisolide	Inhaled Corticosteroids

Main System Use

SABA

It binds specifically to beta2-adrenergic receptors located on the smooth muscle cells that line the airways in the lungs

Pearls

- **SE : jitteriness, increased HR, tremors**
- **Assess lung function regularly**
- **Caution patients with cardiovascular conditions**
- **Anaphylaxis : hives, swelling, difficulty breathing**

Main System Use

Inhaled Corticosteroids :

Targets and inhibits various inflammatory mediators, including cytokines and chemokines, which play a central role in the inflammatory response of the airways

Pearls

- **SE: jitteriness, increased HR, tremors. hoarseness**
- **Increase risk of oral candidiasis**
- **Contraindication: acute exacerbations, mycobacterial infections**

RESPIRATORY

COPD

Definition of the disease

COPD stands for Chronic Obstructive Pulmonary Disease, and it refers to a group of progressive respiratory disorders that cause airflow obstruction and breathing difficulties. The two main conditions included in COPD are chronic bronchitis and emphysema, often coexisting in affected individuals. COPD is a leading cause of morbidity and mortality globally, and it has a significant impact on an individual's respiratory function and overall health. Early diagnosis and a comprehensive approach to management are essential to optimize outcomes for individuals with COPD.

Brand Name	Generic Name	Classification
Ventolin, ProAir, AccuNeb, Vospire, Salbutamol, Proventil	Albuterol	Short-Acting Beta-Agonist (SABA)
Serevent, Fordil, Perforomist, Arcapta Neohaler	Salmeterol, Formoterol Indacaterol	Long acting beta agonist **(LABA)**
Atrovent, Spiriva Cogentin, Benadryl, Ditropan	Ipratropium, Tiotropium, Scopolamine, Benztropine, Diphenhydramine, Oxybutynin	Anticholinergic*

Main System Use

Anticholinergics

Blocking the action of acetylcholine, a neurotransmitter in the parasympathetic nervous system

Pearls

- **SE: dry mouth, constipation, blurry vision, urinary retention**
- **Hydration is necessary**
- **Caution elderly**
- **Contraindicated: GI disorders, glaucoma, urinary retention, cognitive impairment**

RESPIRATORY

Chronic Bronchitis

Definition of the disease

Chronic Bronchitis is a type of chronic obstructive pulmonary disease (COPD) characterized by inflammation of the bronchial tubes, which carry air to and from the lungs. This inflammation leads to persistent coughing and increased production of mucus over an extended period, typically for at least three months per year and for multiple consecutive years.

Brand Name	Generic Name	Classification
Ventolin, ProAir, AccuNeb, Vospire, Salbutamol, Proventil	Albuterol	Short-Acting Beta-Agonist (SABA)

Main System Use

SABA

Binds specifically to beta2-adrenergic receptors located on the smooth muscle cells that line the airways in the lungs

Pearls

- SE: jitteriness, increased HR, tremors
- Assess lung function regularly
- Caution patients with cardiovascular conditions
- Anaphylaxis: hives, swelling, difficulty breathing

RESPIRATORY

Pneumonia

Definition of the disease

Pneumonia is an inflammatory condition affecting the air sacs in one or both lungs, typically caused by infection. The air sacs, also known as alveoli, can become filled with pus or other liquid, leading to symptoms such as cough, fever, and difficulty breathing. Pneumonia can range from mild to severe and can affect people of all ages, but it can be particularly serious in older adults, young children, and individuals with weakened immune systems. Pneumonia can range from mild cases that can be treated at home to severe cases requiring hospitalization. Prompt diagnosis and appropriate treatment are crucial to prevent complications and ensure a successful recovery.

Brand Name	Generic Name	Classification
Zithromax, Zithromax Z-Pak, Zmax, AzaSite, and Zithromax,TRI-PAK, **Levaquin**	**Azithromycin,** Levofloxacin	**Macrolide/** Flouroquinolone
Amoxil, Moxatag, Trimox	Amoxicillin	Penicillin
Augmentin, Augmentin ES-600, and Augmentin XR	**Amoxicillin / Clavulanate**	**Penicillin (Beta - lactamase)**

Main System Use

Amoxicillin: interfering with the synthesis of the bacterial cell wall

Augmentin: enhances amoxicillin making it more effective against a broader range of bacteria

Pearls

- **Monitor for allergies/skin rash**
- Increase fluid intake
- Monitor kidney fxn (amox)
- Monitor Renal fxn (aug)

Main System Use

Fluoroquinolones : targets bacterial DNA gyrase and topoisomerase IV, enzymes responsible for DNA replication and repair

Pearls

- Monitor for Tendon Injury
- **Avoid in elderly if possible**
- Educate on prolonged sun exposure
- Caution potential CNS side effects
- **Prolonged QT intervals**

Pertussis

Definition of the disease

Pertussis, commonly known as whooping cough, is a highly contagious respiratory infection caused by the bacterium Bordetella pertussis. It primarily affects the respiratory tract, particularly the airways, and is characterized by severe coughing fits that often end in a distinctive whooping sound as the affected person tries to inhale. Due to the highly contagious nature of pertussis and the potential severity of the disease, early diagnosis and vaccination are critical preventive measures. Timely treatment with antibiotics can also help control the spread of the disease and mitigate its impact, especially in vulnerable populations such as infants.

Brand Name	Generic Name	Classification
Ery-tab, Eryc EryPed, Illotycin	Erythromycin	Macrolide

Main System Use

Erythromycin :
Involving its ability to inhibit bacterial protein synthesis

Pearls

- **SE: Nausea/ Diarrhea/ Skin Reactions**
- **Increase Risk of Cdiff**
- Avoid Alcohol
- Renal and Hepatic function monitoring
- **No: Cardiac Arrhythmias/ Long QT Syndrome**

ENDOCRINE

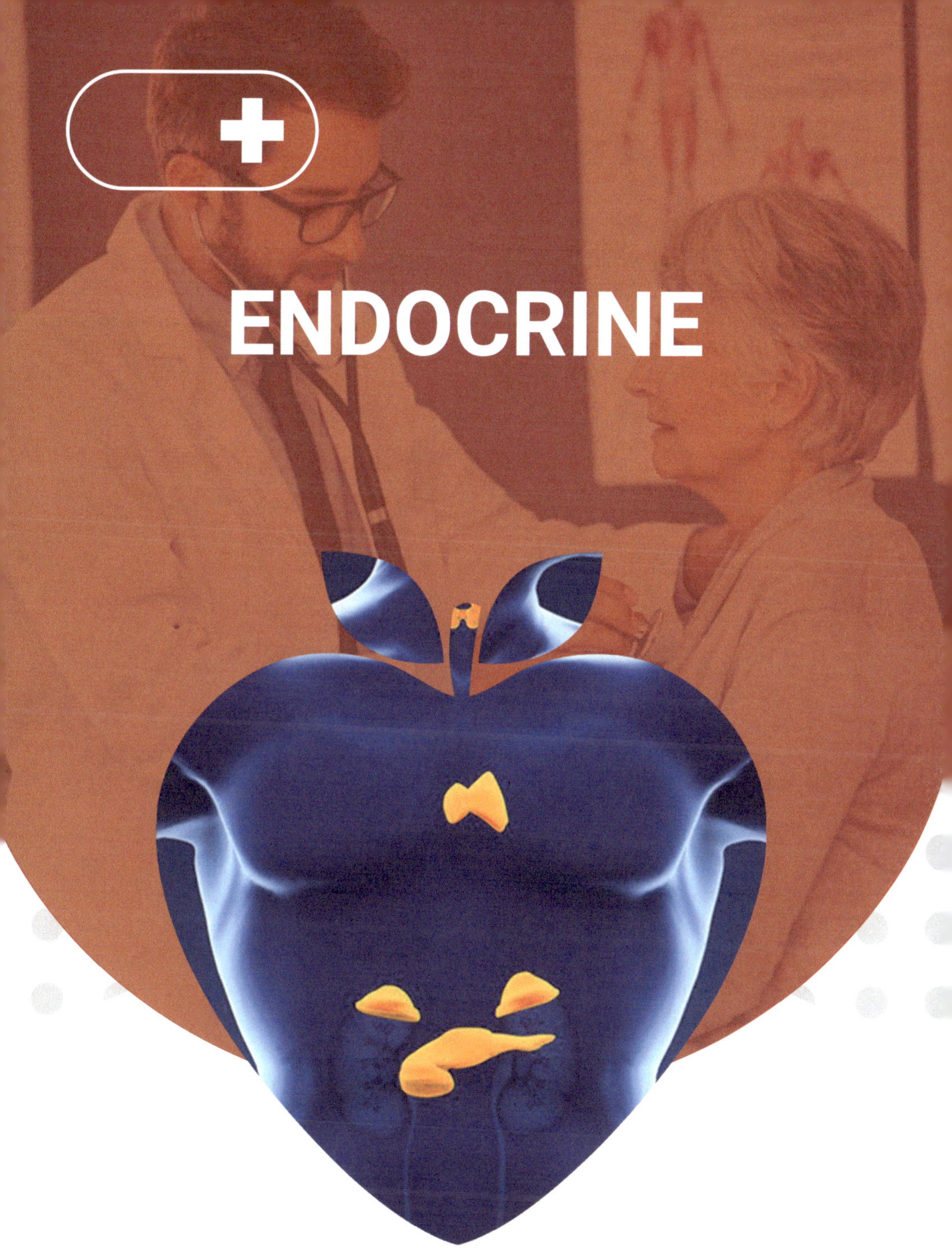

Latrina Walden™
Exam Solutions

ENDOCRINE

Hypothyroidism

Definition of the disease

Hypothyroidism is a medical condition characterized by an underactive thyroid gland, which leads to insufficient production and release of thyroid hormones. The thyroid gland, located in the front of the neck, plays a crucial role in regulating various metabolic processes in the body by producing hormones, primarily thyroxine (T4) and triiodothyronine (T3).

Brand Name	Generic Name	Classification
Synthroid, Tirosint, Levoxyl, Unithroid, and Levo-T	Levothyroxine	Thyroid Hormones

Main System Use

Levothyroxine

Replaces thyroid hormone that your body does not make.

Controls– not cures

Pearls

- Tums or Iron need to be taken 4 hrs prior
- Lifelong Therapy
- Overdose = hyperthyroidism
- Monitor TSH levels regularly
- Assess for chest pain, SOB, flushing, wheezing
- Caution: sucralfate/ antacids/ PPI

ENDOCRINE

Hyperthyroidism

Definition of the disease

Hyperthyroidism is a condition in which the thyroid gland becomes overactive and produces an excessive amount of thyroid hormones, leading to a range of symptoms and potential health issues. Methimazole works by inhibiting the thyroid gland's ability to produce thyroid hormones, specifically by interfering with the synthesis of thyroxine (T4) and triiodothyronine (T3). This helps to reduce the levels of thyroid hormones in the body, effectively managing the symptoms and complications associated with hyperthyroidism, including rapid heart rate, weight loss, and other related issues. Methimazole is often prescribed to normalize thyroid hormone levels and improve the health of individuals with hyperthyroidism.

Brand Name	Generic Name	Classification
Synthroid, Tirosint, Levoxyl, Unithroid, and Levo-T	Levothyroxine	Thyroid Hormones

Main System Use

Inhibiting the thyroid gland's ability to produce thyroid hormones

Pearls

- Monitor labs
- PTU is preferred in 1st trimester of pregnancy
- Monitor liver & WBC fxn
- Iodine rich foods can interfere
- HR/weight/energy levels are to be monitored
- Hepatoxicity/ leukopenia/ n/ v can occur (PTU)

ENDOCRINE

Diabetes

Definition of the disease

Diabetes is a chronic medical condition characterized by elevated levels of glucose (sugar) in the blood. This condition arises when the body is unable to effectively produce or use insulin, a hormone that regulates blood sugar and facilitates the uptake of glucose by cells for energy. There are two main types of diabetes: Type 1 diabetes and Type 2 diabetes. Effective management and control of diabetes require ongoing monitoring, adherence to treatment plans, and regular medical follow-ups. It is a condition that individuals can live with by making informed lifestyle choices and working closely with healthcare providers to optimize their health.

Brand Name	Generic Name	Classification
Glucophage, Glumetza, Riomet, Glucophage XR, and Fortamet	**Metformin**	Biguanide
Invokana Farxiga Jardiance	Canagliflozin, Dapagliflozin, and Empagliflozin	Sodium-Glucose Co-Transporter-2 **(SGLT2)**
DiaBeta, Glynase, or Micronase	Glipizide, Glyburide, Glimepiride	Sulfonylureas
Trulicity	Dulaglutide	**GLP-1**
Ozempic	Semaglutide	**GLP-1**

ENDOCRINE

Diabetes

Main System Use

Metformin : decrease the production of glucose by the liver and increase the sensitivity of peripheral tissues (muscles and fat) to insulin
SGLT2 : inhibit the SGLT-2 protein in the kidneys, which is responsible for reabsorbing glucose from the urine back to the bloodstream
GLP-1 : helps regulate blood sugar by increasing insulin secretion, slowing down gastric emptying, and reducing glucagon secretion
Sulfonylureas : stimulate the pancreas to release more insulin

Pearls

Metformin :

- **Monitor kidney fxn**
- **GI side effects**
- Monitor B12 levels
- **Lactic Acidosis Awareness**

SGLT-2's :

- Increased UTI's
- Dehydration and Hypotension Awareness
- Ketoacidosis Awareness
- Electrolyte Imbalance (K+)

Pearls

GLP-1's:

- **Rotation of injection site**
- GI side effects
- Monitor blood glucose levels
- Hypoglycemic Awareness
- Medication Storage
- Pancreatic Risk
- **Weight Loss**

Pearls

Sulfonylureas

- **Hypoglycemic Risk**
- **Alcohol Interaction**
- Assess Renal Function
- Monitor blood glucose levels

GASTROENTEROLOGY

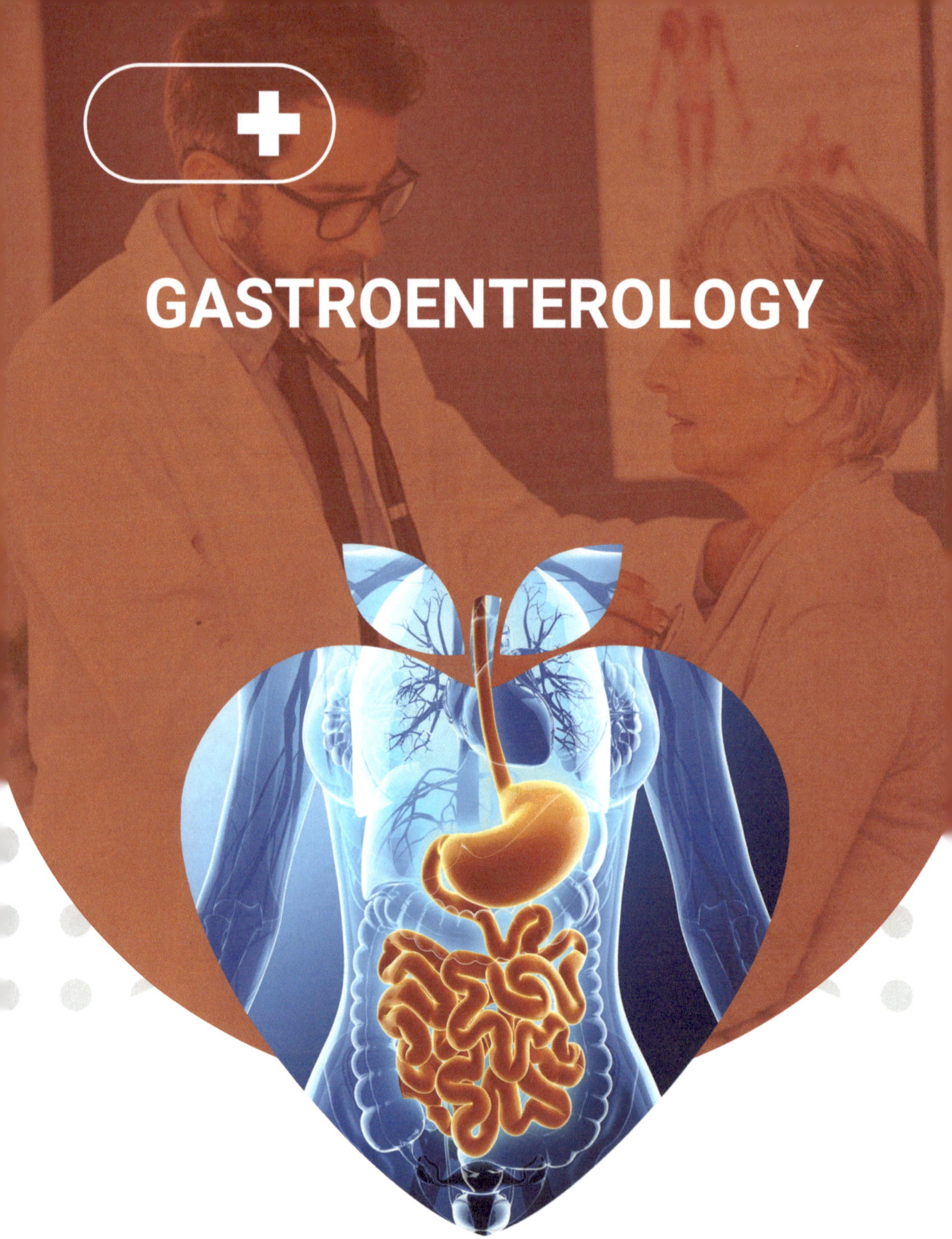

Latrina Walden™
Exam Solutions

GASTROENTEROLOGY

GERD

Definition of the disease

GERD stands for Gastroesophageal Reflux Disease. It is a chronic condition where stomach acid consistently flows back into the esophagus, causing irritation and inflammation. The lower esophageal sphincter (LES), a ring of muscle between the esophagus and stomach, usually acts as a valve that opens to allow food into the stomach and closes to prevent stomach acid from flowing back into the esophagus. In individuals with GERD, the LES is weakened or relaxes inappropriately, allowing stomach acid to reflux into the esophagus.

Brand Name	Generic Name	Classification
Nexium, Nexium IV, Nexium Packet	**Esomeprazole**	**PPI**
Zegerid OTC, Zegerid, OmePPi, and Prilosec OTC	**Omeprazole**	**PPI**
Protonix	Pantoprazole	**PPI**
Aciphex	Pantoprazole	**PPI**

Main System Use

Inhibits the enzyme H+/K+-ATPase (proton pump) in the gastric parietal cells, which is responsible for the final step in the production of gastric acid

Pearls

- Carefully evaluate long-term use
- GI SE
- **Vitamin/ Mineral Deficiencies**
- **Potential drug Interactions**
- **Bone Health**
- C-diff Risk
- Diet and Lifestyle Modification

GASTROENTEROLOGY

GERD

Definition of the disease

GERD is a chronic condition that requires ongoing management and treatment to relieve symptoms and prevent complications. Individuals experiencing symptoms suggestive of GERD should seek evaluation and guidance from a healthcare professional. We only use H2 blockers on an intermittent (PRN) basis typically.

Brand Name	Generic Name	Classification
Zantac	Ranitidine	**H2 blocker**
Tagamet	Cimetidine	**H2 blocker**
Pepcid	Famotidine	**H2 blocker**

Main System Use

These medications work by blocking the action of histamine on the H2 receptors in the stomach lining. This action reduces the production of stomach acid.

Pearls

- Evaluate duration of use
- Evaluate renal and liver function
- Beware for b12 deficiency
- Encourage lifestyle modifications

GENITOURINARY

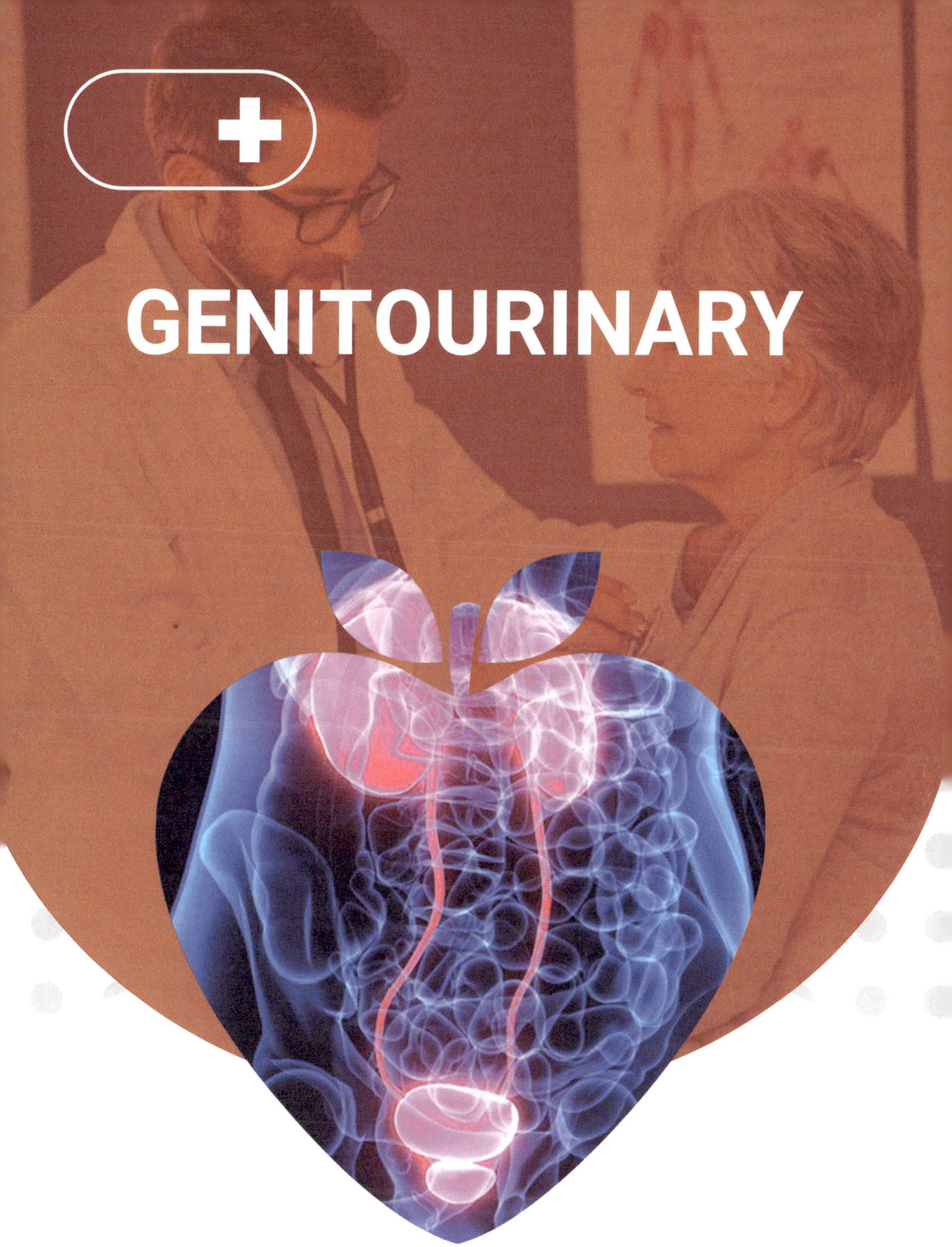

Latrina Walden™
Exam Solutions

GENITOURINARY

Urinary Tract Infection /Pyelonephritis

Definition of the disease

A urinary tract infection (UTI) is a bacterial infection that affects any part of the urinary system, which includes the kidneys, bladder, ureters (tubes that connect the kidneys to the bladder), and the urethra (the tube through which urine exits the body). UTIs are common and can range from mild to severe. UTIs are common, especially in women, and prompt diagnosis and treatment are important to prevent complications.

Pyelonephritis is a type of urinary tract infection (UTI) that specifically involves inflammation and infection of the kidneys. It is often a result of bacteria, typically Escherichia coli (E. coli), ascending from the lower urinary tract to the kidneys. Pyelonephritis can be acute or chronic and is considered a more severe form of UTI.

Brand Name	Generic Name	Classification
Bactrim DS, Sulfatrim, and Bactrim	Sulfamethoxazole / Trimethoprim	Sulfonamide
Cetraxal, Cipro XR, Otiprio, Cipro inD5W, and Ci loxan	**Ciprofloxacin**	Fluoroquinolone
Furadantin, Macrodantin	**Nitrofurantoin**	**Macrobid**
Omincef, Keflex, Suprax	Cefaclor, **Cefdinir**, Cefixime, Cephradine, **Cephalexin; (all oral)**	Cephalosporins

Urinary Tract Infection /Pyelonephritis

Main System Use

Macrobid : acts by damaging bacterial DNA

Fluoroquinolones : targets bacterial DNA gyrase and topoisomerase IV, enzymes responsible for DNA replication and repair

Cephalosporins : disrupts bacterial cell wall synthesis, leading to cell lysis and death

Bactrim : impairs the production of DNA and RNA, which inhibits bacterial growth and reproduction

Pearls

Macrobid :
- Take with food
- Increase water intake

Fluoroquinolones :
- Monitor for Tendon Injury
- **Avoid in elderly if possible**
- Educate on prolonged sun exposure
- Caution potential CNS side effects

Pearls

Oral Cephalosporins:
- Monitor for allergic reaction
- Increased C-diff risk

Bactrim :
- **Monitor for skin reaction (SJ)***
- Increased risk for hyperkalemia
- Increase water intake
- Caution potential CNS side effects

GENITOURINARY

Benign Prostatic Hyperplasia

Definition of the disease

Benign Prostatic Hyperplasia (BPH), also known as prostate gland enlargement, is a common condition that affects aging men. BPH is characterized by the non-cancerous enlargement of the prostate gland, which surrounds the urethra and is situated just below the bladder. As the prostate enlarges, it can squeeze or partially block the urethra, leading to various urinary symptoms. While BPH is not cancerous, it can significantly impact quality of life due to urinary symptoms. Men experiencing symptoms suggestive of BPH should consult with a healthcare professional for an accurate diagnosis and appropriate management.

Brand Name	Generic Name	Classification
Propecia, Propecia Pro- Pak, and Proscar	**Finasteride**	**5-Alpha-Reductase Inhibitors**
Hytrin	Terazosin	**Alpha Blockers**
Flomax	**Tamsulosin**	**Alpha Blockers**

Main System Use

5 alpha reductase :
inhibiting the conversion of testosterone to DHT, these medications decrease the levels of DHT in the body

Alpha blockers :
targets alpha-adrenergic receptors in smooth muscle tissues, leading to relaxation of these muscles

Pearls

5 alpha reductase :

- Educate that it will take time
- **Libido/Erectile dysfunction SE**
- **Monitor for urinary output**
- SE education – gynecomastia
- Monitor liver function

Alpha Blockers:

- **Blood pressure monitoring**
- Assess urinary output
- Educate on medication timing
- **SE – headache/ dizziness/ fatigue**
- Monitor tapering

NOSE/THROAT

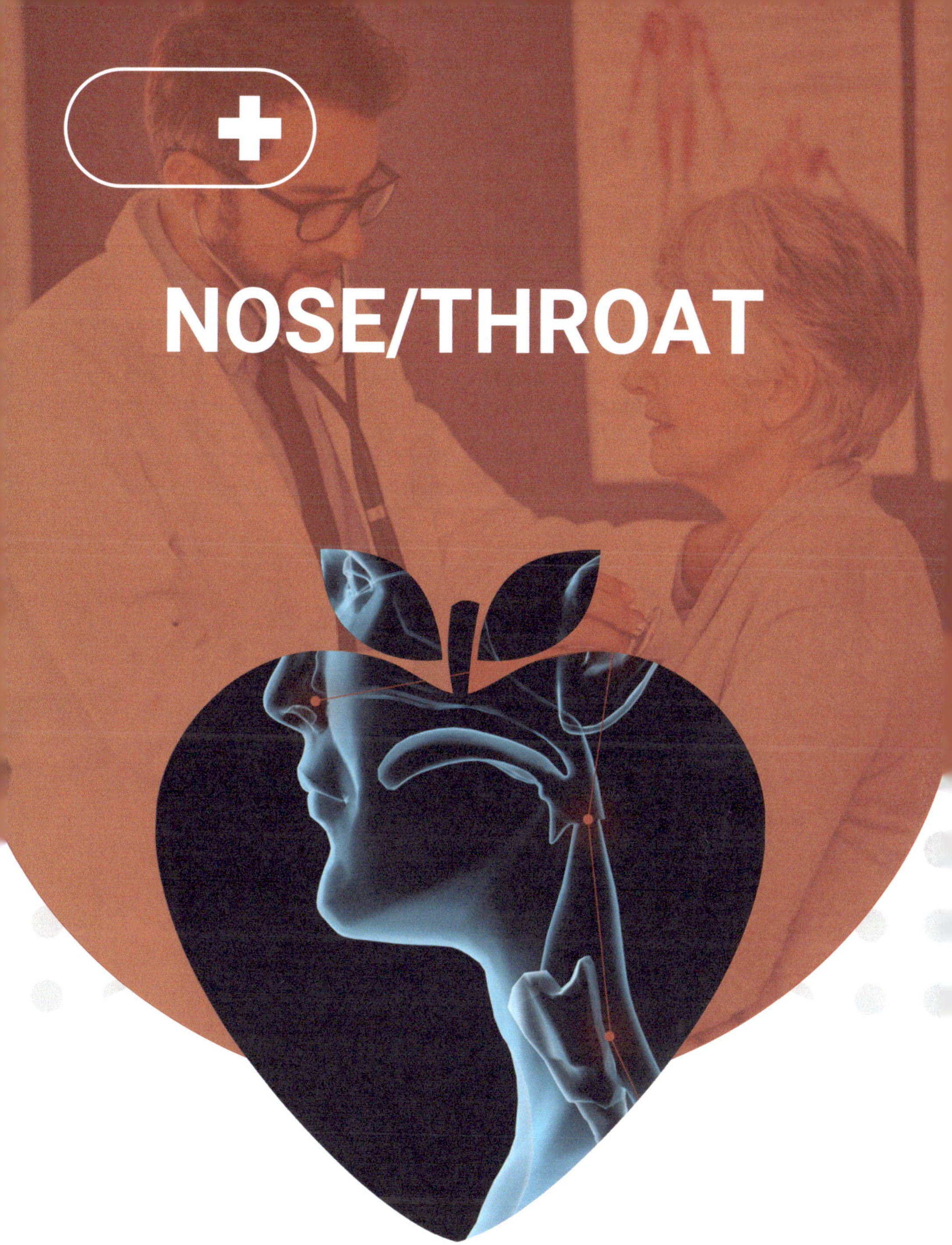

Latrina Walden™
Exam Solutions

Pharyngitis/ Strep Throat

Definition of the disease

Pharyngitis is the medical term for inflammation of the pharynx, which is the back of the throat. This condition is commonly referred to as a sore throat. Pharyngitis can be caused by various factors, including viral or bacterial infections, irritants, or environmental factors. Pharyngitis is a common condition and is often a self-limiting illness. However, bacterial causes, particularly streptococcal infections, may require antibiotic treatment to prevent complications and reduce the risk of transmission to others. Individuals with persistent or severe symptoms should seek medical evaluation for proper diagnosis and management.

Brand Name	Generic Name	Classification
Penicillin V, Penicillin G, Bicillin, Veetids, Beepen VK	**Penicillin**	Penicillin

Main System Use

Penicillin:
targets and bind to enzymes known as penicillin-binding proteins (PBPs), which are involved in the synthesis of the bacterial cell wall

Pearls

- **Monitor for allergies/ skin rash**
- **Assess for allergy**
- Cross-Reactivity: Penicillin and other beta-lactams ex. Cephalosporins
- Monitor renal function

Sinusitis

Definition of the disease

Sinusitis is the inflammation or swelling of the tissues that line the sinuses, which are air-filled cavities in the skull around the nose. This inflammation can cause the sinuses to become blocked, leading to the accumulation of mucus and creating an environment where bacteria or viruses can thrive. While acute sinusitis often resolves on its own or with conservative measures, chronic sinusitis may require more comprehensive management, and persistent or severe symptoms should be evaluated by a healthcare professional. Individuals with recurrent or chronic sinusitis may benefit from consultation with an ear, nose, and throat (ENT) specialist.

Brand Name	Generic Name	Classification
Augmentin, Augmentin ES-600, and AugmentinXR	Amoxicillin / Clavulanate	Penicillin (Beta - lactamase)
Amoxil, Moxatag, Trimox	Amoxicillin	Penicillin
Fluticasone, Budesonide	Corticosteroids	Steroids

Main System Use

Amoxicillin : interfering with the synthesis of the bacterial cell wall

Augmentin : enhances amoxicillin making it more effective against a broader range of bacteria

Pearls

- **Monitor for allergies/ skin rash**
- Increase fluid intake
- Monitor kidney fxn (amox)
- Monitor Renal fxn (aug)

Allergic Rhinitis

Definition of the disease

Allergic rhinitis, commonly known as hay fever, is an allergic reaction that occurs when the immune system overreacts to allergens in the air, particularly airborne particles like pollen, dust mites, mold spores, pet dander, or certain particles from cockroaches. When individuals with allergic rhinitis come into contact with these allergens, it triggers an inflammatory response in the nasal passages, leading to a range of symptoms. While there is no cure, effective management strategies, including medications and allergen avoidance, can help control symptoms and improve daily functioning.

Brand Name	Generic Name	Classification
Flonase Nasacort	Fluticasone Propionate Triamcinolone Acetonide	Intranasal Corticosteroid
Nasalcrome	Cromolyn	Mast cell stabilizers

Main System Use

Mast Cell Stabilizers : functions by preventing the release of histamine and other inflammatory mediators from mast cells

Intranasal Corticosteroids : these work by reducing inflammation in the nasal passages and other affected areas of the respiratory tract

Pearls

Mast Cell Stabilizers :

- Use before allergy exposure
- SE – nasal irritation/sneezing
- Assess response
- Hypersensitivity awareness

Intranasal Corticosteroids :

- Teach Proper Application
- Rinse and Spit
- Contraindications

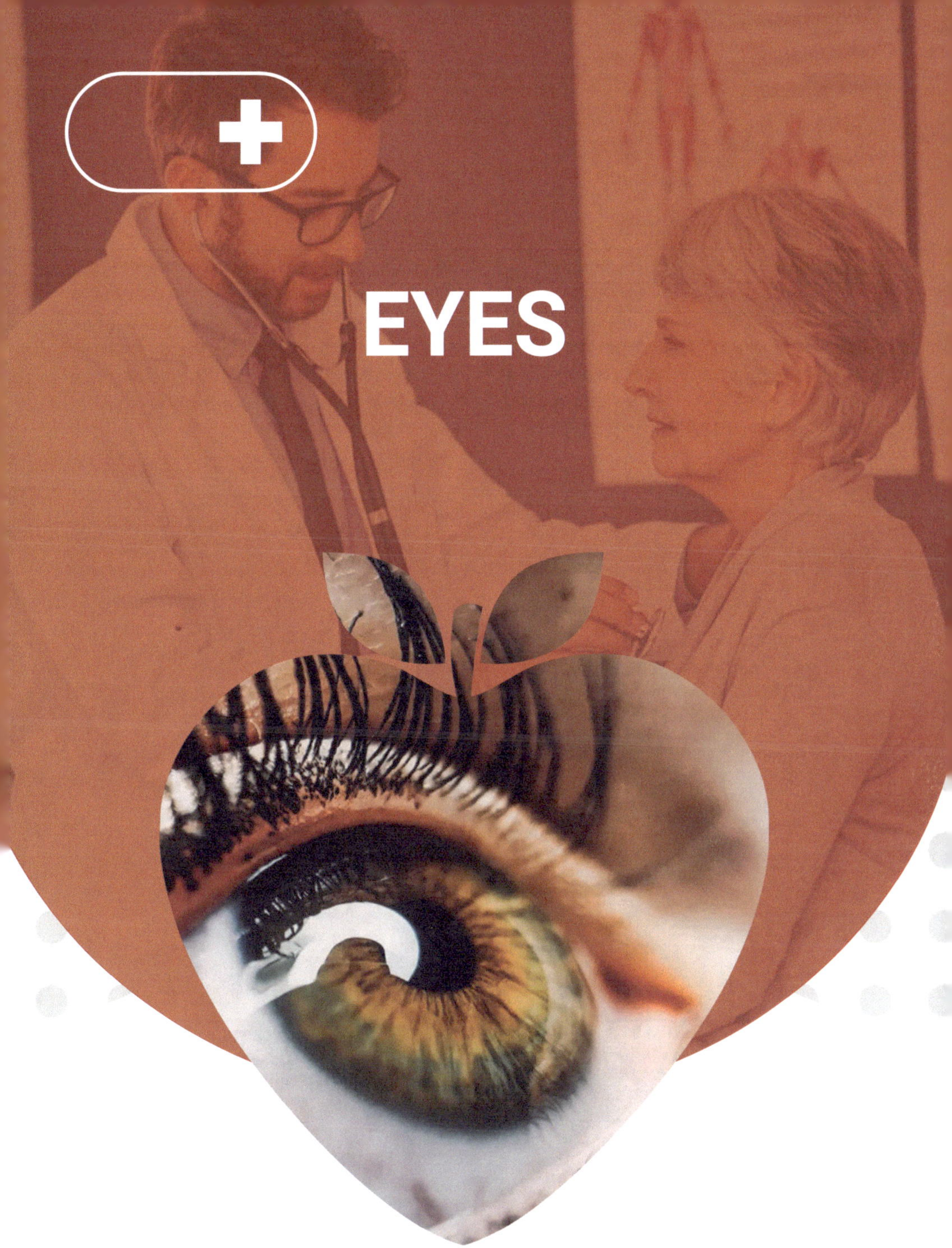

EYES

Latrina Walden™
Exam Solutions

Glaucoma

Definition of the disease

Glaucoma is a group of eye conditions that damage the optic nerve, which is crucial for transmitting visual information from the eye to the brain. The damage is often associated with elevated intraocular pressure (IOP), but glaucoma can also occur with normal or low IOP. If left untreated, glaucoma can lead to irreversible vision loss and blindness. Early detection and treatment are essential for managing glaucoma and preventing vision loss. Since the condition often progresses without noticeable symptoms, routine eye examinations are critical, especially for individuals at higher risk

Brand Name	Generic Name	Classification
Timoptic-xe, Istalol, EYES Timoptic, Betimol, and Timoptic Ocudose (PF)	**Timolol** Maleate	**Beta - Blockers**
Xalatan	Latanoprost	**Prostaglandin** Analog

Main System Use

Beta Blockers:
blocking beta-adrenergic receptors in the ciliary body, beta-blockers decrease the production of aqueous humor, leading to lower intraocular pressure

Prostaglandin:
analogs relax the smooth muscle in the uveoscleral pathway, allowing more aqueous humor to flow out of the eye, thus reducing intraocular pressure

Pearls

Beta Blockers:
- Infection control
- Medication adherence
- **Cardiovascular monitoring**
- Reactions in the eye: burning/ stinging

Prostaglandins :
- **SE – redness/ eyelash changes/ skin darkening/. eye discharge (crusting)**
- **Iris darkening**
- Caution breastfeeding

Conjunctivitis

Definition of the disease

Conjunctivitis, commonly known as pink eye, is the inflammation of the conjunctiva—the thin, clear tissue that covers the white part of the eye and lines the inner surface of the eyelids. This inflammation can be caused by various factors, including infections, allergies, irritants, or underlying medical conditions. Conjunctivitis is a common and often self- limiting condition. However, appropriate management depends on determining the underlying cause.

Brand Name	Generic Name	Classification
Poly-Rx	**Polymyxin B**	Polymyxins
Cipro/Cetraxal/ Proquin Floxin	Ciprofloxacin **Ofloxacin**	Fluoroquinolones
Zithromax, Zithromax Z-Pak, Zmax, AzaSite, and Zithromax TRI-PAK	**Azithromycin**	Macrolide

Conjunctivitis

Main System Use

Polymyxin B is an antibiotic with a primary action that involves disrupting the integrity of bacterial cell membranes

Fluoroquinolones : targets bacterial DNA gyrase and topoisomerase IV, enzymes responsible for DNA replication and repair

Azithromycin : inhibit the growth of bacteria by interfering with their protein synthesis

Pearls

Polymyxin B :

- **Monitor Renal Function** Hypersensitivity awareness
- **Monitor for neurotoxicity (paresthesia)**
- **SE-GI**

Azithromycin :

- May increase warfarin toxicity
- Report diarrhea/blood or pus in stool
- **SE: colitis, pain, diarrhea, nausea, Stevens-Johnsons syndrome, Angioedema**

Fluoroquinolones :

- Monitor for Tendon Injury
- Avoid in elderly if possible
- Educate on prolonged sun exposure
- Caution potential CNS side effects

EYES

Blepharitis

Definition of the disease

Blepharitis is a common and chronic inflammation of the eyelids, particularly at the base of the eyelashes. It can affect people of all ages and is often associated with a dysfunction of the oil glands located near the base of the eyelashes. Blepharitis can be uncomfortable, but it is usually not contagious and doesn't typically cause permanent damage to eyesight.

Brand Name	Generic Name	Classification
Ery-tab, Eryc EryPed, Illotycin	**Erythromycin**	Macrolide
Neosporin / Polyspori / Baciguent	Bacitracin	**Fluoroquinolones**

Main System Use

Erythromycin :
bprimary mechanism of action involving its ability to inhibit
bacterial protein synthesis through binding of ribosomes

Bacitracin :
binds to a molecule called bactoprenol, which plays a crucial role in transporting the building blocks of the cell wall (such as peptidoglycans) to the site of cell wall synthesis on the bacterial cell membrane

Pearls

Beta Blockers:

- E: Nausea/Diarrhea/Skin Reactions
- Increase Risk of Cdiff
- Avoid Alcohol
- Renal and Hepatic function monitoring
- No: Cardiac Arrhythmias/ Long QT Syndrome

Bacitracin :

- **Infection Control**
- No : Intranasal/ Intraocular usage

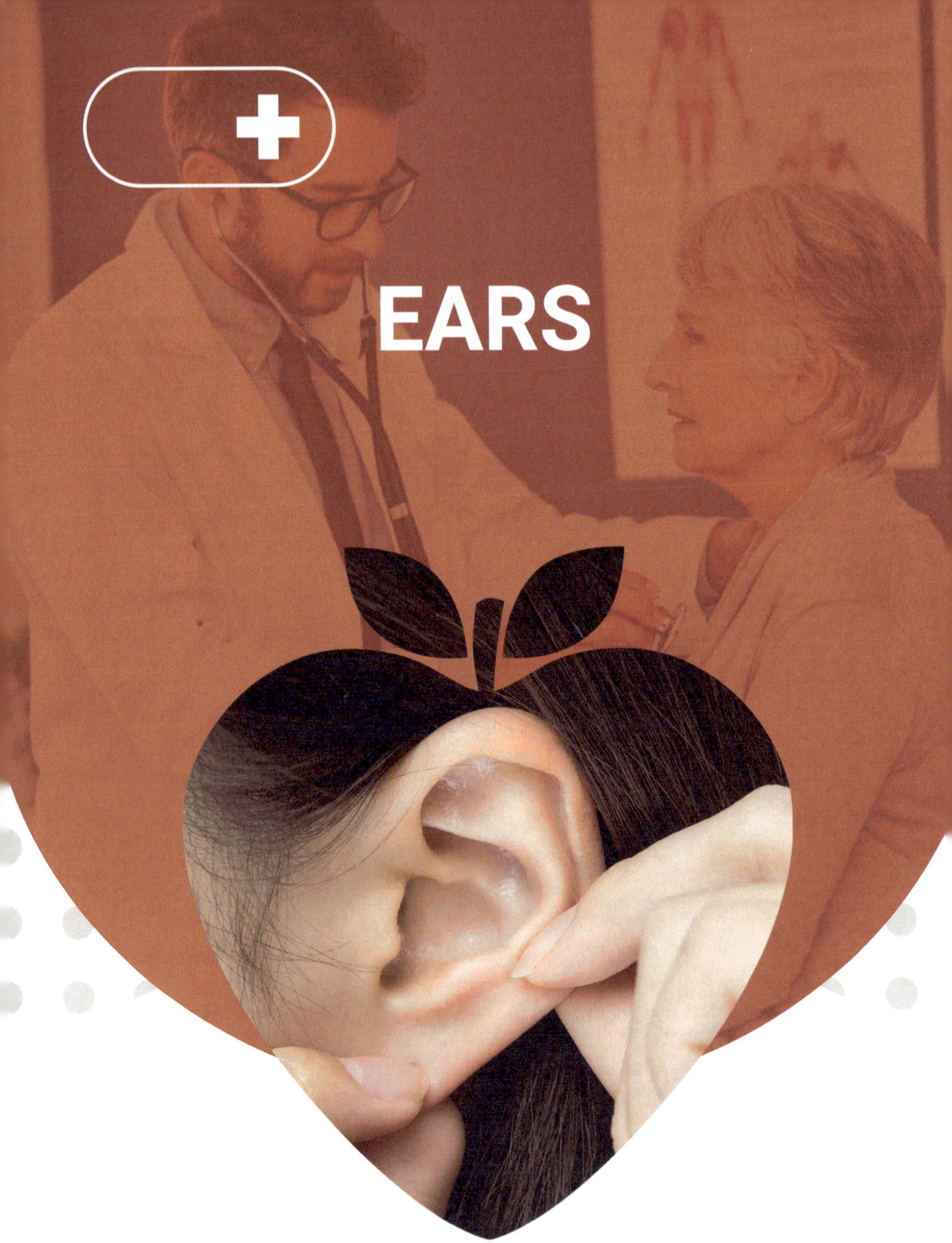

EARS

Latrina Walden™
Exam Solutions

EARS

Acute Otitis Media

Definition of the disease

Acute Otitis Media (AOM) is a common ear infection that occurs when there is inflammation and infection in the middle ear. The middle ear is the space located behind the eardrum, and it contains the small bones responsible for transmitting sound vibrations. AOM is often seen in children but can also affect individuals of any age. Acute Otitis Media is a common condition, and many cases resolve on their own or with appropriate treatment.

Brand Name	Generic Name	Classification
Moxatag et. Al.	Amoxicillin	Penicillin
Omnicef	Cefdinir	Cephalosporin
Augmentin, Augmentin ES-600, and Augmentin XR	Amoxicillin / Clavulanate	

Main System Use

Amoxicillin : interfering with the synthesis of the bacterial cell wall
Augmentin : enhances amoxicillin making it more effective against a broader range of bacteria

Pearls

- Increase fluid intake
- Monitor kidney fxn (amox)
- Monitor Renal fxn (aug)
- **Monitor for allergies/ skin rash**

Main System Use

Cephalosporins :
disrupts bacterial cell wall synthesis, leading to cell lysis and death

Pearls

- **Monitor for allergic reaction**
- Increased C-diff risk

Otitis Externa

Definition of the disease

Otitis externa, commonly known as swimmer's ear, is an inflammation or infection of the external ear canal, which is the tube that extends from the outer ear to the eardrum. This condition is often associated with water exposure, and it can cause discomfort, pain, and swelling. Otitis externa is a common condition and is usually not serious if promptly and appropriately treated. In severe or persistent cases, or if there are signs of complications such as cellulitis or abscess formation, medical attention should be sought. Individuals with diabetes or weakened immune systems may be at a higher risk of complications and should consult a healthcare provider if they suspect otitis externa.

Brand Name	Generic Name	Classification
Poly-Rx	**Polymyxin B**	Polymyxin
Cipro/Cetraxal/ Proquin Floxin	Ciprofloxacin **Ofloxacin**	Fluoroquinolones
Pred Forte, Alrex, Lotemax	**Corticosteroid drops**	Steroids

Main System Use

Polymyxin B:
is an antibiotic with a primary action that involves disrupting the integrity of bacterial cell membranes

Fluoroquinolones :
targets bacterial DNA gyrase and topoisomerase IV, enzymes responsible for DNA replication and repair

Corticosteroid drops :
ophthalmologic anti-inflammatory agent

Pearls

Polymyxin B:

- **Monitor Renal Function**
- Hypersensitivity awareness
- **Monitor for neurotoxicity (paresthesia)**
- **SE-GI**

Fluoroquinolones :

- Monitor for Tendon Injury
- **Avoid in elderly if possible**
- Educate on prolonged sun exposure
- Caution potential CNS side effects

Aphthous Ulcer/ Stomatitis

Definition of the disease

Aphthous Ulcers, commonly known as Canker Sores, are painful, shallow sores that form on the mucous membranes inside the mouth. These ulcers are typically round or oval-shaped and have a white or yellowish center with a red border. They can develop on the inside of the lips, cheeks, under the tongue, or on the floor of the mouth. Aphthous ulcers are a common oral condition and are usually benign, not being associated with serious health issues. While aphthous ulcers can be uncomfortable, they are generally harmless and not contagious. If ulcers are persistent, recurrent, or associated with other concerning symptoms, it's advisable to seek advice from a healthcare professional or a dentist for a proper evaluation and guidance on management.

Brand Name	Generic Name	Classification
Benadryl	Liquid Diphenhydramine	Antihistamines
Lidocaine Viscous Lidoderm, Recticare	**Viscous Lidocaine**	Local anesthetic
Medrol (Pro), Deltasone (Pro), Cortef (Pro), Dexamethasone Intensol	Corticosteroids	Glucocorticoids

Main System Use

Liquid Diphenhydramine : main action is to block the effects of histamine

Viscous Lidocaine : Temporarily numb or relieve pain in the mucous membranes

Corticosteroid : inhibiting the production of inflammatory cytokines, including interleukins and tumor necrosis factor (TNF)

Pearls

Polymyxin B:

- Sedation likely
- **Caution pediatric and elderly**
- Consider cough/gag reflex
- Risk of Aspirations
- Risk of difficulty breathing

MENS AND WOMENS HEALTH REVIEW AND STIs

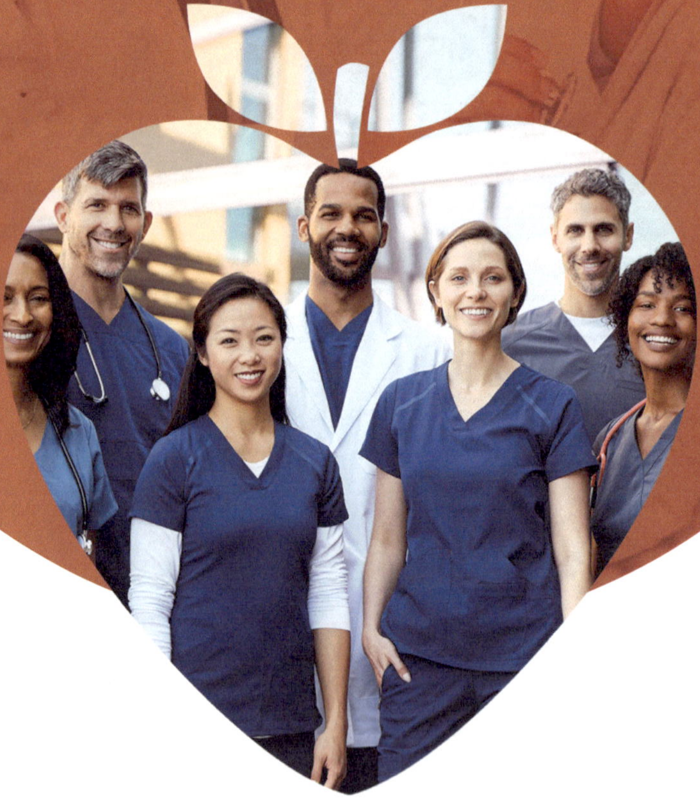

Latrina Walden™
Exam Solutions

Candida Vaginitis

Definition of the disease

Candida vaginitis, also known as vaginal yeast infection or vulvovaginal candidiasis, is a common fungal infection that affects the female genital area. It is primarily caused by the overgrowth of the fungus Candida, most commonly Candida albicans. Candida is a type of yeast that is normally present in small amounts in the vagina, but certain factors can lead to an imbalance, resulting in an infection. Candida vaginitis is a common and treatable condition. Most women experience relief with appropriate antifungal treatment.

Brand Name	Generic Name	Classification
Diflucan	Fluconazole	Antifungal s
Lotrimin, Monistat	Clotrimazole	Antifungal

Main System Use

Fluconazole & Clotrimazole : works by disrupting the cell membranes of fungi, thereby inhibiting their growth and multiplication by disrupting cell membrane growth

Pearls

Fluconazole:

- Headache/ nausea/ vomiting
- Check liver function
- Avoid alcohol
- Proper storage
- Avoid overuse due to resistance

Clotrimazole :

- Importance of hygiene/. hand hygiene
- Avoid mouth/ eye contact
- Report burning/ redness/ swelling

Vaginal Atrophy

Definition of the disease

Vaginal Atrophy, also known as Atrophic Vaginitis or Genitourinary Syndrome of Menopause (GSM), is a condition that occurs when the vaginal tissues become thinner, drier, and less elastic due to a decrease in estrogen levels, often associated with menopause. While it is most commonly seen in postmenopausal women, it can also affect women during other life stages when estrogen levels decline, such as during breastfeeding or certain cancer treatments. Vaginal atrophy is a common condition associated with hormonal changes, particularly during and after menopause.

Brand Name	Generic Name	
Estradiol Topical	Topical Estrogen	Estrogen Hormones

Main System Use

Estradiol :
It exerts its effects by binding to estrogen receptors found in various tissues throughout the body

Pearls

- Monitor for SE : breast tenderness, mood changes, blood clots
- Monitor bone health

Genital Warts

Definition of the disease

Genital Warts, also known as Condylomata Acuminata, are a sexually transmitted infection (STI) caused by certain strains of the Human PapillomaVirus (HPV).
HPV is a group of viruses that can infect the genital and anal areas, as well as the mouth and throat. Genital warts are one of the most common manifestations of HPV infection. While treatment can remove visible warts, it may not eliminate the underlying HPV infection. Regular medical check-ups, HPV vaccination, and safe sex practices are crucial for preventing and managing genital warts and reducing the risk of associated complications.

Brand Name	Generic Name	Classification
n/a	Acetic Acid	Organic Acid

Main System Use

It has an astringent effect on the tissues. This causes the genital warts, which are made up of thickened, keratinized skin cells, to become dehydrated and take up the acetic acid solution

Pearls

- No: eyes, mouth, open wounds or broken skin
- **May induce anxiety**
- Be concerned about patient comfort
- Proper dilution
- **Caution skin irritation and burns**

Chlamydia

Definition of the disease

Chlamydia is a common sexually transmitted infection (STI) caused by the bacterium Chlamydia Trachomatis. It is one of the most prevalent bacterial STIs globally and can affect both men and women. Chlamydia is primarily transmitted through sexual contact, including vaginal, anal, or oral sex with an infected partner. Chlamydia is a curable infection, and early detection and treatment are essential to prevent complications and reduce the risk of transmission. Individuals at risk for chlamydia should engage in regular STI screenings and practice safe sex behaviors to protect their sexual health.

Brand Name	Generic Name	Classification
Zithromax, Zithromax Z-Pak, Zmax, AzaSite, and Zithromax TRI-PAK	Azithromycin	Macrolide
Monodox, Doxy-100, Targadox, Oracea, Acticlate, Avidoxy, Morgidox, Doryx MPC, Mondoxyne	Doxycycline	Tetracycline

Main System Use

Azithromycin :
inhibits the growth of bacteria by interfering with their protein synthesis

Doxycycline :
main mechanism of action involves interfering with bacterial protein synthesis, thereby inhibiting bacterial growth and reproduction

Pearls

Azithromycin :
- May increase warfarin toxicity
- Report diarrhea/ blood or pus in stool
- **SE: colitis, pain, diarrhea, nausea, Stevens-Johnsons syndrome, Angioedema**

Doxycycline :
- SE: severe rash, anaphylaxis, respiratory distress
- Contraindicated for pregnancy (2nd trimester) and children<8yrs
- Discoloration of teeth and impaired bone growth
- **Check liver function**
- Myasthenia Gravis

Herpes

Definition of the disease

Herpes is a viral infection caused by the Herpes Simplex Virus (HSV). There are two main types of herpes simplex virus: HSV-1 and HSV-2. While both types can cause oral and genital herpes infections, they are generally associated with different areas of the body. Herpes is a lifelong infection, and while treatment can manage symptoms and reduce the frequency of outbreaks, there is no cure. Prevention strategies, including safe sex practices and antiviral medications, can help reduce the risk of transmission.

Brand Name	Generic Name	Classification
Zovirax	Acyclovir	Anti-Viral
Valtrex	Valacyclovir	Anti-Viral

Main System Use

Acyclovir and. Valacyclovir :

inhibits viral replication by interfering with the synthesis of viral DNA

Pearls

- Do not use in neonates
- Caution in patients with renal impairment
- Adequate hydration necessary

Bacterial Vaginosis/ Trichomoniasis

Definition of the disease

Bacterial vaginosis (BV) is a common vaginal infection caused by an imbalance in the natural bacteria that normally inhabit the vagina. In a healthy vagina, there is a delicate balance between beneficial bacteria (such as Lactobacillus) and other microorganisms. When this balance is disrupted, bacterial vaginosis can occur.

Trichomoniasis, often referred to as "trich," is a sexually transmitted infection (STI) caused by the single-celled protozoan parasite Trichomonas Vaginalis. This parasitic infection primarily affects the urogenital tract, including the vagina in women and the urethra in both men and women.

Brand Name	Generic Name	Classification
Flagyl /Metrogel	**Metronidazole**	Antifungal
Cleocin, Clindagel, Dalacin	**Clindamycin**	Lincosamide

Bacterial Vaginosis/ Trichomoniasis

Main System Use

Flagyl:
Disruption of DNA synthesis in certain microorganisms, leading to the inhibition of their growth and replication

Clindamycin :
It works by binding to the 50S ribosomal subunit of bacterial ribosomes, which are essential for protein production in bacterial cells.
This interference with protein synthesis disrupts bacterial growth and replication

Pearls

- **Avoid alcohol**
- Avoid in 1st trimester
- **Monitor liver function**
- GI upset(metallic, n/v, diarrhea)
- Headache/dizziness/dry mouth
- Can increase yeast infections
- Monitor for leukopenia and Thrombocytopenia

Clindamycin

- **Check for cross allergies**
- Monitor for GI upset
- **Increased risk of Cdiff**
- Avoid Alcohol
- **No: hx of pseudomembranous colitis**
- Renal and Hepatic monitoring

Syphilis

Definition of the disease

Syphilis is a Sexually Transmitted Infection (STI) caused by the bacterium Treponema Pallidum. It can manifest in various stages, each with distinct symptoms and potential complications if left untreated. Syphilis is primarily transmitted through sexual contact, including vaginal, anal, or oral sex, as well as through close skin-to-skin contact with syphilis sores.

Brand Name	Generic Name	Classification
Bicillin	Penicillin G	PCN

Main System Use

interference with bacterial cell wall synthesis, ultimately leading to bacterial cell lysis and death

Pearls

- Assess for allergy
- Cross-Reactivity: Penicillin and other beta-lactams
  - ex. Cephalosporins
- Monitor renal function

PCOS

Definition of the disease

Polycystic Ovary Syndrome (PCOS) is a common hormonal disorder that affects individuals with ovaries, typically during their reproductive years. PCOS is characterized by a combination of symptoms related to hormonal imbalances and metabolic dysfunction. The exact cause of PCOS is not fully understood, and it can manifest differently among individuals. PCOS is a heterogeneous condition, meaning that it can vary widely among individuals. Treatment approaches are tailored to address specific symptoms and individual goals, whether they involve regulating menstrual cycles, managing symptoms of hyperandrogenism, addressing metabolic concerns, or supporting fertility.

Brand Name	Generic Name	Classification
Aldactone	Spironolactone	Potassium sparing diuretic
Glucophage, Glumetza, Riomet, Glucophage XR, and Fortamet	Metformin	Biguanide

Main System Use

Metformin :
primary role is to manage insulin resistance and androgen excess in the context of PCOS

Spironolactone :
regulate the balance of electrolytes (sodium and potassium) and fluids in the body, especially by reducing sodium and water retention while sparing potassium. Its anti-androgenic properties are also crucial in managing conditions characterized by excessive androgens

Pearls

Metformin :

- **Monitor kidney fxn**
- **GI side effects**
- Monitor B12 levels
- **Lactic Acidosis Awareness**

Spironolactone :

- **Hyperkalemia**
- Orthostatic Hypotension
- Dietary considerations (K+ rich foods)
- **Monitor renal function**

Acute Prostatitis

Definition of the disease

Acute Prostatitis is an inflammation of the prostate gland that typically develops suddenly and is characterized by symptoms of pain, discomfort, and systemic signs of infection. The prostate is a small, walnut-shaped gland located below the bladder and in front of the rectum, and it plays a role in the production of semen. Prompt diagnosis and treatment of acute prostatitis are crucial to prevent complications and promote a full recovery. If left untreated, acute prostatitis can progress to chronic prostatitis or lead to the development of abscesses in the prostate.

Brand Name	Generic Name	Classification
Cetraxal, Cipro XR, Otiprio, Cipro inD5W, and Ci loxan	**Ciprofloxacin**	Fluoroquinolone
Levaquin	Levofloxacin	**Macrolide**

Main System Use

Fluoroquinolones :
targets bacterial DNA gyrase and topoisomerase IV, enzymes responsible for DNA replication and repair

Pearls

Fluoroquinolones :

- Monitor for Tendon Injury
- **Avoid in elderly if possible**
- Educate on prolonged sun exposure
- Caution potential CNS side effects
- **Prolonged QT intervals**

NEUROLOGY

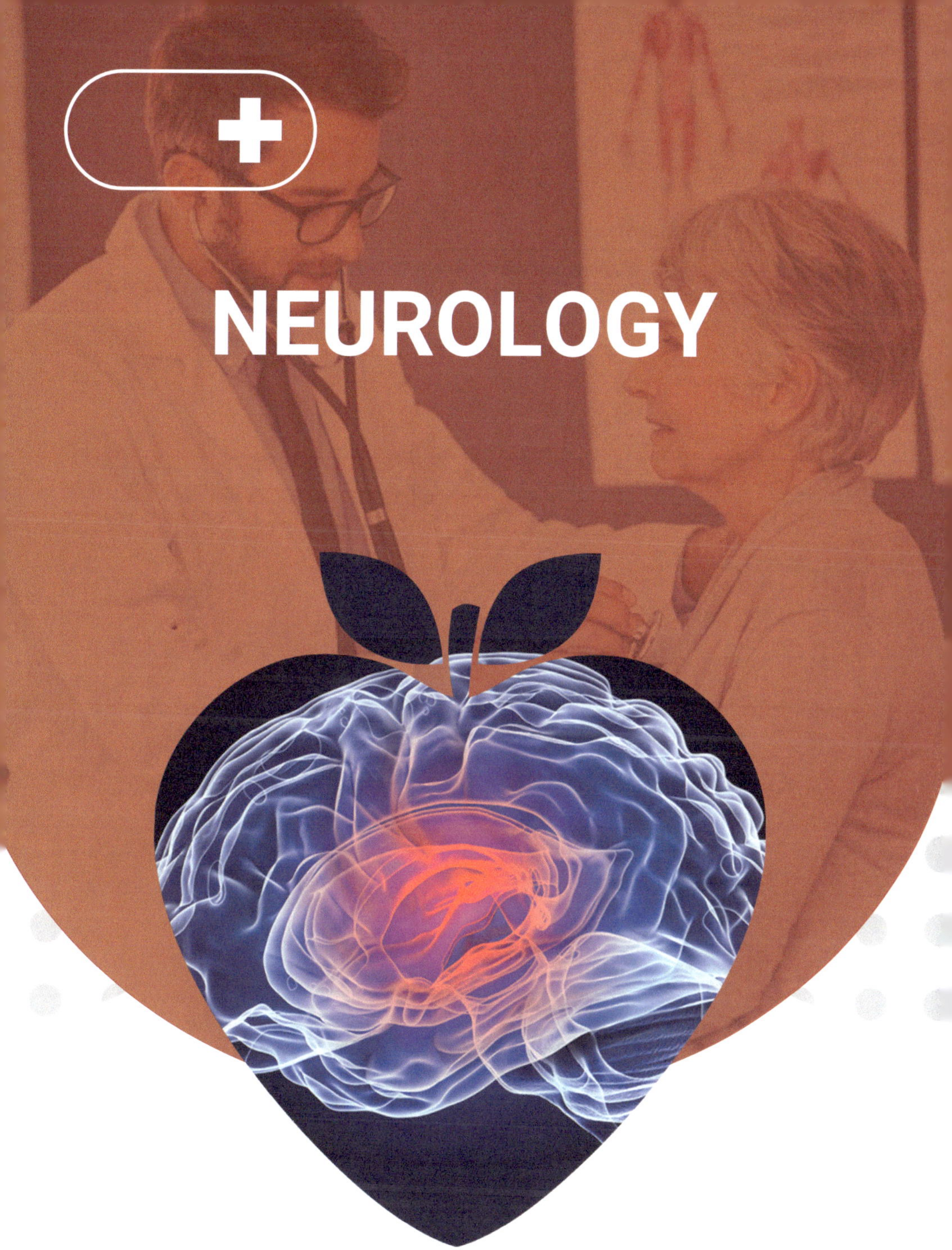

Latrina Walden™
Exam Solutions

NEUROLOGY

Migraine Headaches

Definition of the disease

Migraine Headaches are a type of headache characterized by recurrent, intense, throbbing pain, usually on one side of the head. Migraines are often accompanied by other symptoms, and they can significantly affect daily life.

Brand Name	Generic Name	Classification
Inderal, Inderal LA, Inderal XL, Hemangeol	**Propranolol**	**Beta Blocker**
Imitrex, Alsuma, and Sumavel DosePro	**Sumatriptan**	5-HTI receptor agonists

Main System Use

Propranolol :
Blocks the effects of adrenaline (epinephrine) and other stress-related hormones on the body

Sumatriptan :
is a selective serotonin receptor agonist that binds to the receptors in the walls of blood vessels in the brain causing vasoconstriction.
It also inhibits the release of pro-inflammatory neuropeptides that are involved in the transmission of pain signals

Pearls

Propranolol :

- **Contraindicated in heart blocks, HF and bradycardia unless***
- **Avoid in asthma/ COPD patients**
- Can mask signs of hypoglycemia
- Monitor for Orthostatic Hypotension

Sumatriptan :

- **No –CVA/ HTN/ PVD/ Ischemic Heart Disease**
- Rebound Headaches can occur

NEUROLOGY

Cluster Headaches

Definition of the disease

Cluster headaches are a type of primary headache disorder characterized by severe, recurrent headaches that occur in clusters or groups. These headaches are known for their distinctive pattern of occurring in cyclical patterns or "clusters," typically lasting for weeks to months, followed by periods of remission. Cluster headaches are considered one of the most severe forms of headache. Cluster headaches can significantly impact a person's quality of life, and managing them effectively often requires a combination of acute and preventive treatments tailored to the individual's specific situation

Brand Name	Generic Name	Classification
Verelan, Verelan PM, Calan SR, and Calan	Verapamil	Calcium Channel Blocker
Imitrex, Alsuma, and Sumavel DosePro	Sumatriptan	5-HTI receptor agonists

Main System Use

Calcium Channel Blockers :
Blocking the movement of calcium ions into cardiac and smooth muscle cells

Sumatriptan :
is a selective serotonin receptor agonist that binds to the receptors in the walls of blood vessels in the brain causing vasoconstriction. It also inhibits the release of pro-inflammatory neuropeptides that are involved in the transmission of pain signals

Pearls

Calcium Channel Blockers :

- No – HF/ Heart blocks/ Cardiogenic Shock
- Monitor Blood Pressure
- Monitor Electrolyte Levels (K+ and Ca+2)

Sumatriptan :

- **No –CVA/ HTN/ PVD/ Ischemic Heart Disease**
- Rebound Headaches can occur

Headaches

Definition of the disease

Headaches are a common condition characterized by pain or discomfort in the head, scalp, or neck. They can vary in intensity, duration, and underlying causes. Headaches can be primary or secondary, depending on whether they are the main health problem or a symptom of another condition. Tension-Type Headaches - These are the most common type of primary headache and are often described as a constant band-like pressure around the head.

Brand Name	Generic Name	Classification
Elavil or Endep	Amitriptyline	Tricyclic Antidepressant

Main System Use

Inhibits the reuptake of serotonin and norepinephrine in the brain. Meaning, it increases the levels of these neurotransmitters in the synaptic cleft, which may affect pain perception and transmission

Pearls

- **Avoid MAOI's**
- Avoid those with MI's or Arrythmias
- **Be vigilant for SI**
- Sedation may occur

NEUROLOGY

Korsakoff Syndrome

Definition of the disease

Korsakoff syndrome, also known as Korsakoff's psychosis, is a chronic memory disorder caused by severe deficiency of thiamine (vitamin B1), often associated with long-term heavy alcohol consumption. Thiamine is essential for the proper functioning of the brain, and its deficiency can lead to neurological complications. Korsakoff syndrome is considered a form of alcohol-related brain damage, and its development is associated with chronic alcohol misuse, malnutrition, and thiamine deficiency. It underscores the importance of a balanced and nutritious diet, particularly in individuals with a history of alcohol dependence or other risk factors for thiamine deficiency.

Brand Name	Generic Name	Classification
Thiamine	Vitamin B1	Vitamin

Main System Use

Converted into its active form, thiamine pyrophosphate (TPP), within the body; TPP acts as a cofactor for several enzymes involved in the citric acid cycle (Krebs cycle) and other metabolic pathways. This coenzyme is involved in several biochemical reactions, including those related to carbohydrate metabolism and energy production.

Pearls

- **Caution those with renal impairment**
- Be vigilant of alcohol

NEUROLOGY

Essential Tremor

Definition of the disease

Essential tremors are a neurological disorder characterized by involuntary, rhythmic trembling or shaking of a part of the body, most commonly the hands. It is one of the most common movement disorders, and while the exact cause is not well understood, it is believed to have a genetic component. Essential tremor is distinct from other tremor disorders, such as Parkinson's disease.

Brand Name	Generic Name	Classification
Inderal	**Propranolol**	**Beta-blocker**

Main System Use

Propranolol :
Blocking the effects of adrenaline (epinephrine) and other stress-related hormones on the body

Pearls

Propranolol :

- **Contraindicated in heart blocks, HF and bradycardia**
- **Avoid in asthma/ COPD patients**
- Can mask signs of hypoglycemia
- Monitor for Orthostatic Hypotension

NEUROLOGY

Temporal Arteritis

Definition of the disease

Temporal Arteritis, also known as giant cell arteritis (GCA), is a vasculitis—a group of disorders characterized by inflammation of blood vessels. Temporal arteritis specifically involves the medium to large arteries, particularly those around the temples. This condition predominantly affects individuals who are over the age of 50.

Brand Name	Generic Name	Classification
Deltasone, Prednicot, Prednisone Intensol	Oral Prednisone	Corticosteroids

Main System Use

Prednisone :
Inhibiting the production of inflammatory cytokines, including interleukins and tumor necrosis factor (TNF)

Pearls

- **Monitor glucose control**
- **Monitor bone health**
- Possible increase risk for infections
- **Taper appropriately**
- Can increase intraocular pressure
- Pt with hx of mood disorder monitor

PEDIATRICS

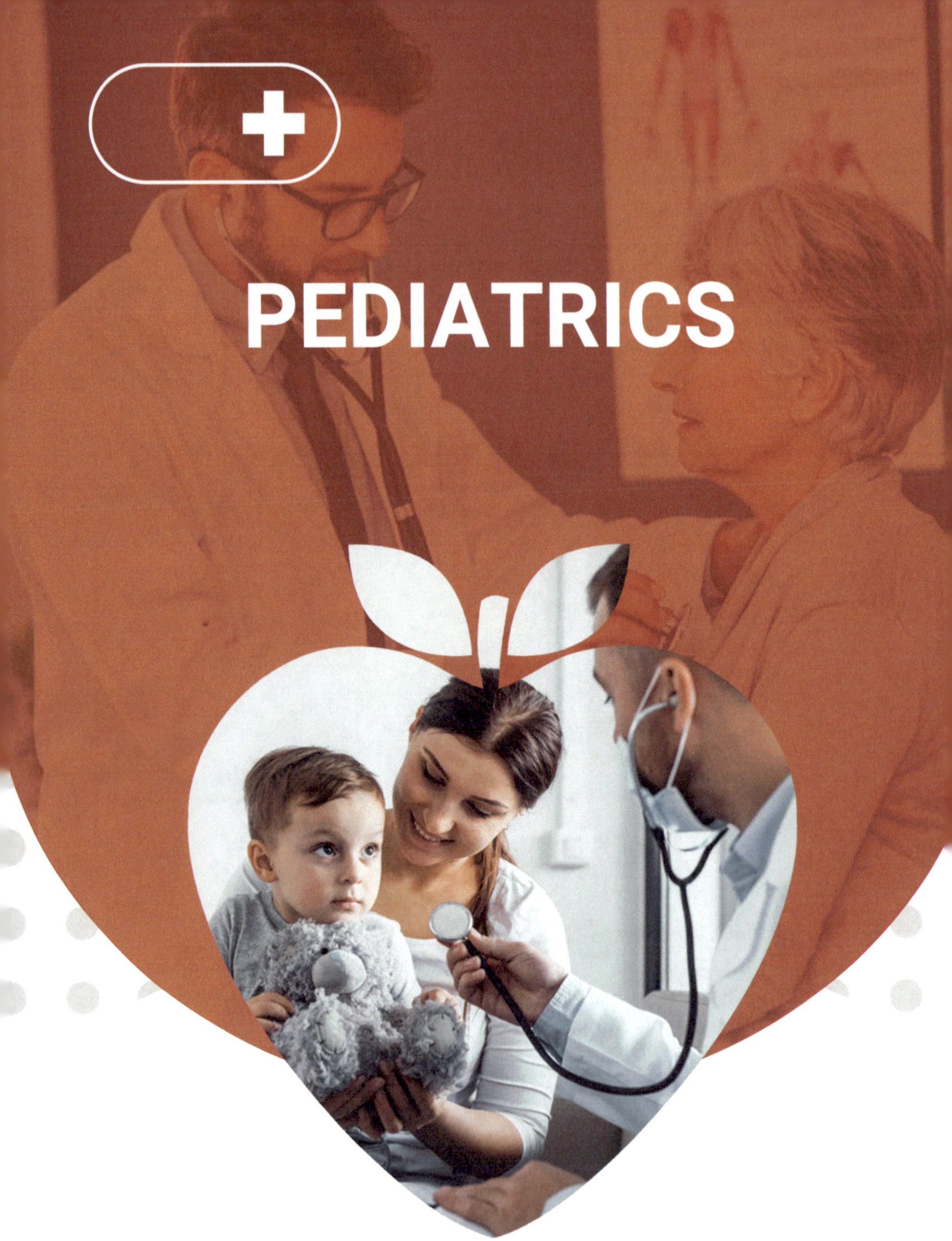

Latrina Walden™
Exam Solutions

Treatment of ADHD

Definition of the disease

Attention-Deficit/ Hyperactivity Disorder (ADHD) is a neurodevelopmental disorder that commonly begins in childhood but can persist into adolescence and adulthood. ADHD is characterized by persistent patterns of inattention, hyperactivity, and impulsivity that can interfere with daily functioning and development.

Brand Name	Generic Name	Classification
Adderall IR	Amphetamine or Dextroamphetamine	Stimulants
Vyvanse	Lisdexamfetamine	Stimulants
Strattera	Atomoxetine	Non-stimulants
Ritalin	Methylphenidate	Stimulants

Treatment of ADHD

Main System Use

Adderall and Vyvanse : Dextroamphetamine stimulates the release of norepinephrine and dopamine from nerve cells into the synaptic cleft (the gap between nerve cells)

Strattera : It inhibits the reuptake of norepinephrine in the brain, leading to increased levels of this neurotransmitter in the synaptic cleft (the gap between nerve cells)

Ritalin : Methylphenidate stimulates the release of dopamine and norepinephrine from nerve cells into the synaptic cleft (the gap between nerve cells)

Pearls

- **Avoid in patients with cardiovascular disease**
- Caution for those with Hyperthyroidism
- **Psych Evals are needed**
- Monitor BP/ HR
- Monitor weight
- **Monitor for SI**
- Be aware of appetite suppression
- Avoid those with Cardiovascular disease/ arteriosclerosis
- Hyperthyroidism
- **Monitor weight/BP/ HR**

PSYCHIATRIC

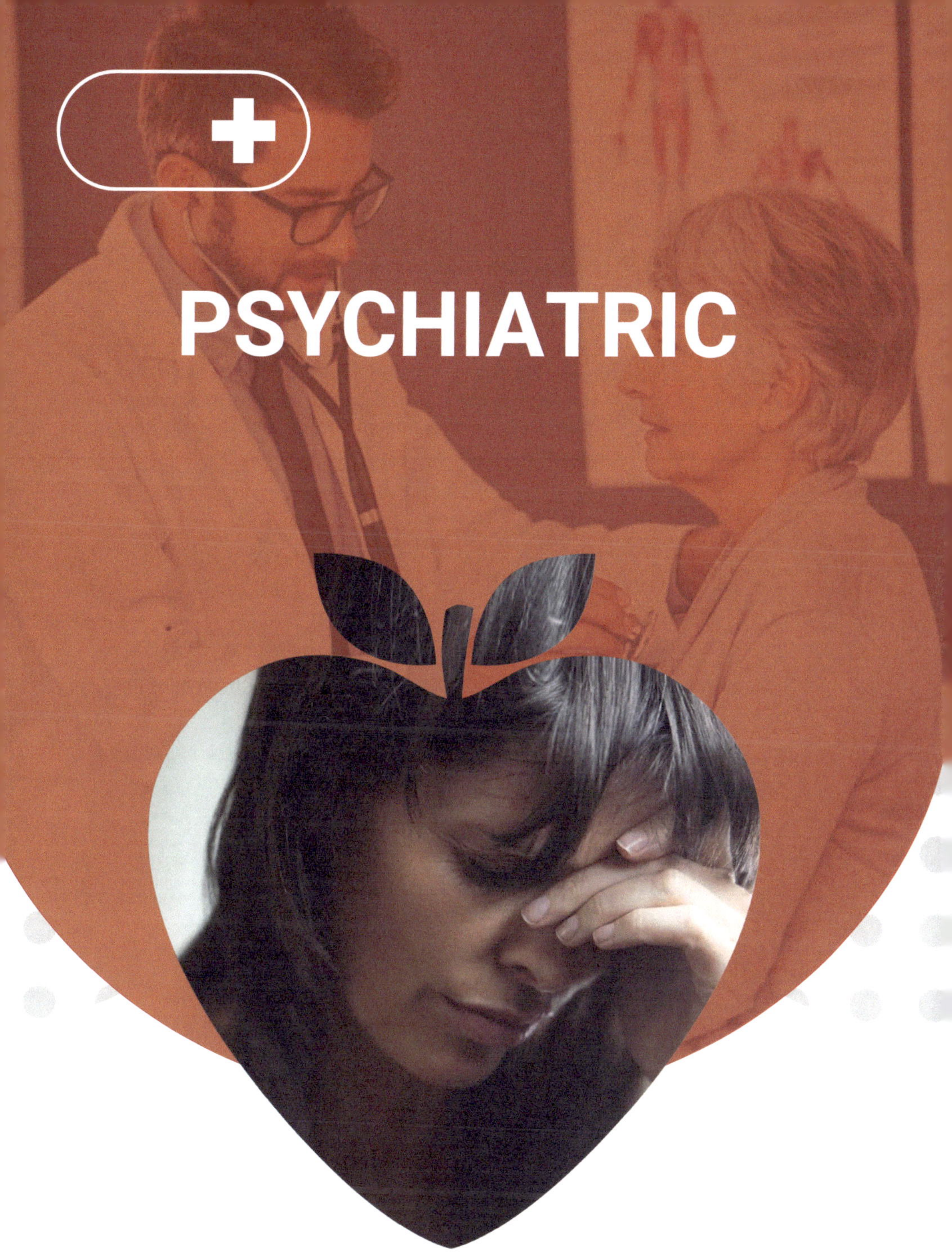

Latrina Walden™
Exam Solutions

PSYCHIATRIC

Psychiatric

Definition of the disease

Psychiatric medications refer to drugs prescribed for the treatment of mental health conditions and disorders. These medications are designed to alleviate symptoms, manage symptoms over the long term, or address underlying imbalances in brain chemistry. Psychiatric medications are prescribed by healthcare professionals, typically psychiatrists or other providers like FNP's and PMHNPs, after a thorough evaluation of the individual's symptoms, medical history, and overall health. Regular monitoring, adjustment of dosages, and addressing potential side effects are essential components of psychiatric medication management.

Brand Name	Generic Name	Classification
Neurontin	Gabapentin	Anticonvulsants
Prozac	**Fluoxetine**	SSRI
Zoloft	Atomoxetine	**SSRI**
Cymbalta	**Duloxetine**	SNRI
Wellbutrin XL, Wellbutrin SR, Forfivo XL, Aplenzin, and Zyban	Bupropion	NORI

Psychiatric

Main System Use

Gabapentin increase the synthesis and release of GABA, which is an inhibitory neurotransmitter in the central nervous system

Fluoxetine inhibit the reuptake of serotonin in the brain

Sertraline prevents the reuptake of serotonin by nerve cells, allowing more serotonin to remain in the synaptic cleft between neurons.

Duloxetine inhibiting serotonin reuptake, duloxetine increases the availability of serotonin in the synapses between nerve cells.

Wellbutrin inhibits the reuptake of both norepinephrine and dopamine in the brain

Pearls

Gabapentin :

- Monitor for SI
- Monitor Renal Function
- **Caution to elderly**
- **Potential Sedation**
- Potential for misuse

Sertraline :

- **Hyponatremia**
- Beware headache, confusion, weakness, seizure, coma
- **Avoid MAOI's**
- **Caution elderly**
- Monitor SI

Fluoxetine :

- **Hyponatremia**
- Avoid with migraine meds
- Avoid with MAOI
- **Avoid abrupt cessation**
- Monitor SI

Duloxetine :

- Avoid MOI's
- Severe Liver Disease
- **Uncontrolled Glaucoma**

Wellbutrin :

- Provide support for smoking
- withdrawal symptoms
- **Seizure risk**
- Monitor BP
- Caution those with eating disorders
- **Contraindicated in hepatic impairment**

PSYCHIATRIC

Benzodiazepines

Definition of the disease

Benzodiazepines are a class of psychoactive drugs that exert their effects on the central nervous system (CNS). These medications have various therapeutic uses, primarily for their anxiolytic (anti-anxiety), sedative, hypnotic (sleep-inducing), anticonvulsant, and muscle relaxant properties. Benzodiazepines work by enhancing the inhibitory effects of a neurotransmitter called gamma-aminobutyric acid (GABA) in the brain. These medications are generally recommended for short-term use in many cases, and alternative treatments may be explored for chronic conditions.

Brand Name	Generic Name	Classification
Xanax	Alprazolam	Benzodiazepines
Ativan	Lorazepam	Benzodiazepines
Valium	Diazepam	Benzodiazepines

Main System Use

Xanax, Valium & Ativan :

Enhances the activity of GABA by binding to specific GABA receptors in the brain

Pearls

- **SE: drowsiness/ dizziness/ impaired coordination**
- Monitor for SI
- Avoid abrupt discontinuation
- Caution elderly
- **No: acute narrow-angle glaucoma/ myasthenia gravis**
- No with opioids

PSYCHIATRIC

Antipsychotics & Mood

Definition of the disease

Antipsychotics, also known as neuroleptics, are a class of medications primarily used to manage symptoms of psychosis. Psychosis is a mental health condition characterized by a disconnection from reality, which may include hallucinations, delusions, disorganized thinking, and impaired insight. Antipsychotic medications work by influencing the activity of neurotransmitters, particularly dopamine, in the brain.

"Mood Medications" is a broad term that can refer to medications used to stabilize or regulate mood in individuals experiencing mood disorders or disturbances. These medications are often prescribed to manage conditions such as depression, bipolar disorder, anxiety disorders, and certain other mood-related conditions. The specific class of mood medication prescribed depends on the nature of the mood disorder and the symptoms exhibited by the individual.

Brand Name	Generic Name	Classification
Zyprexa	Olanzapine	Atypical Antipsychotics
Respiradol	Risperidone	Atypical Antipsychotics
Seroquel	Quetiapine	Atypical Antipsychotics
Lithobid	Lithium	Mood Stabilizer

Main System Use

Zyprexa, Seroquel & Respiradol : Exerts its effects in part by blocking dopamine receptors in the brain. They blocks certain serotonin receptors, specifically the 5-HT2A receptors.

Lithium : Reduce norepinephrine release, which can help stabilize mood and reduce the manic phase of bipolar disorder

Pearls

- Metabolic Monitoring
- Caution elderly
- No: Coma/Seizures
- Prolongs QT interval
- Caution Arrythmias
- Hydration
- Maintain sodium intake (Hyponatremia)
- Monitor kidney and thyroid
- Caution with heart disease

DERMATOLOGY

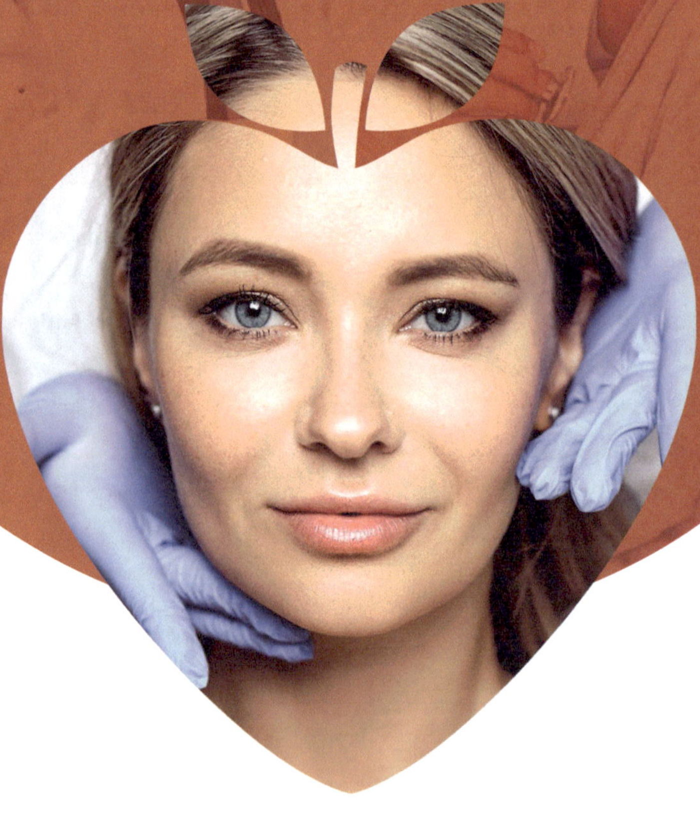

Latrina Walden™
Exam Solutions

DERMATOLOGY

Cellulitis

Definition of the disease

Cellulitis is a common, potentially serious bacterial skin infection characterized by redness, swelling, warmth, and tenderness of the affected area. It occurs when bacteria, most commonly Streptococcus or Staphylococcus, enter the skin through a break or wound, spreading into the deeper layers of the dermis and subcutaneous tissues. Symptoms may include fever, chills, and swollen lymph nodes. Prompt treatment with antibiotics is essential to prevent complications, such as abscesses or the spread of the infection to the bloodstream (sepsis).

Brand Name	Generic Name	Classification
Cleocin, Clindagel, Dalacin	Clindamycin	Lincosamide
Augmentin, Augmentin ES-600, and Augmentin XR	Amoxicillin / Clavulanate	Penicillin
Omnicef, Keflex, Suprax	Cefaclor, Cefdinir, Cefixime, Cephradine, Cephalexin (all oral)	Cephalosporins

Main System Use

Cephalosporins :
Disrupts bacterial cell wall synthesis, leading to cell lysis and death

Augmentin :
Enhances amoxicillin making it more effective against a broader range of bacteria

Clindamycin :
Elt works by binding to the 50S ribosomal subunit of bacterial ribosomes, which are essential for protein production in bacterial cells. This interference with protein synthesis disrupts bacterial growth and replication

Pearls

5 alpha reductase :

- Monitor for allergic reaction
- Increased C-diff risk

Alpha Blockers:

- Monitor for allergies/skin rash
- Increase fluid intake
- Monitor kidney fxn (amox)
- Monitor Renal fxn (aug)

- Check for cross allergies
- Monitor for GI upset
- Increased risk of Cdiff
- Avoid Alcohol
- No: hx of pseudomembranous colitis
- Renal and Hepatic monitoring

DERMATOLOGY

Impetigo

Definition of the disease

Impetigo is a highly contagious bacterial skin infection that primarily affects infants and young children, though it can occur at any age. It is caused by Staphylococcus Aureus or Streptococcus Pyogenes bacteria. The infection typically presents as red sores or blisters on the face, especially around the nose and mouth, as well as on the hands and feet. These sores rupture quickly, oozing and forming a honey-colored crust. Impetigo spreads easily through direct contact with the sores or contaminated items. Treatment typically involves topical or oral antibiotics to clear the infection and prevent its spread.

Brand Name	Generic Name	Classification
Cleocin, Clindagel, Dalacin	Clindamycin	Lincosamide

Main System Use

Binding to isoleucyl-tRNA synthetase leading to the inhibition of protein synthesis in bacteria which means they can't grow and simplify

Pearls

- Do not apply to open wounds
- Caution with pregnancy/breastfeeding
- Avoid contact with eyes or mucous membranes
- SE: rash, itchiness, swelling, severe dizziness,
- difficulty breathing (allergic reactions)
- Hand hygiene

MRSA

Definition of the disease

MRSA (Methicillin-Resistant Staphylococcus aureus) is a type of staph bacterial infection that is resistant to many commonly used antibiotics, including methicillin, making it more challenging to treat. MRSA infections typically manifest as painful, swollen red bumps or abscesses that may be warm to the touch, filled with pus, or accompanied by fever. These infections can occur on the skin but may also affect deeper tissues, joints, or the bloodstream, leading to more severe health complications. MRSA is spread through direct contact with infected wounds or contaminated surfaces, and treatment often requires specific antibiotics that the bacteria have not yet become resistant to. Preventative measures, such as good hygiene and wound care, are essential to limit the spread of MRSA.

Brand Name	Generic Name	Classification
Bactrim DS, Sulfatrim, and Bactrim	Sulfamethoxazole/ Trimethoprim	Sulfonamide
Cleocin, Clindagel, Dalacin	Clindamycin	Lincosamide
Monodox, Doxy-100, Targadox, Oracea, Acticlate, Avidoxy, Morgidox, Doryx MPC, Mondoxyne	Doxycycline	Tetracycline

MRSA

Main System Use

Bactrim
Impairs the production of DNA and RNA, which inhibits bacterial growth and reproduction

Clindamycin
It works by binding to the 50S ribosomal subunit of bacterial ribosomes, which are essential for protein production in bacterial cells. This interference with protein synthesis disrupts bacterial growth and replication.

Doxycycline
Main mechanism of action involves interfering with bacterial protein synthesis, thereby inhibiting bacterial growth and reproduction

Pearls

Bactrim :

- Monitor for skin reaction (SJ)
- Increased risk for Hyperkalemia
- Increase water intake
- Caution potential CNS side effects

Clindamycin :

- Check for cross allergies
- Monitor for GI upset
- Increased risk of Cdiff
- Avoid Alcohol
- No: hx of pseudomembranous colitis
- Renal and Hepatic monitoring
-

Doxycycline :

- SE: severe rash, anaphylaxis, respiratory distress
- Contraindicated for pregnancy (2nd trimester) and children<8yrs
- Discoloration of teeth and impaired bone growth
- Check liver function
- Myasthenia Gravis

PSYCHIATRIC

Cdiff: Clostridium Difficile

Definition of the disease

Clostridium difficile (C. difficile or C. diff) is a spore-forming bacterium that causes inflammation of the colon, known as colitis, primarily resulting in severe diarrhea. It is often associated with recent antibiotic use, which disrupts the balance of healthy bacteria in the gut, allowing C. difficile to proliferate. Symptoms include watery diarrhea, abdominal pain, fever, and, in severe cases, dehydration or life-threatening complications like toxic megacolon. C. difficile infections are highly contagious and can spread through contact with contaminated surfaces or fecal matter. Treatment typically involves specific antibiotics such as vancomycin or fidaxomicin, along with infection control measures to prevent spread in healthcare settings. In recurrent or severe cases, fecal microbiota transplantation (FMT) may be considered.

Brand Name	Generic Name	Classification
Flagyl/ Metrogel	Metronidazole	Antifungal
Vancocin, Vancomycin Hydrochloride, Vancomycin HCl	Vancomycin	Glycopeptide

Main System Use

Flagyl :
Disruption of DNA synthesis in certain microorganisms, leading to the inhibition of their growth and replication

Vancomycin :
High affinity for a specific molecule in the bacterial cell wall called D-Alanine-D-Alanine. It binds to this molecule, preventing the synthesis of the cell wall and weakening its structural integrity

Pearls

Flagyl :

- Avoid alcohol
- Avoid in 1st trimester
- Monitor liver function
- GI upset(metallic, n/v, diarrhea)
- Headache/dizziness/dry mouth
- Can increase yeast infections
- Monitor for leukopenia and thrombocytopenia

Vancomycin :

- Monitor renal function
- Caution red man syndrome
- Caution ototoxicity

DERMATOLOGY

Psoriasis

Definition of the disease

Psoriasis is a chronic autoimmune skin condition characterized by the rapid buildup of skin cells, leading to thickened, red patches covered with silvery-white scales. These patches, or plaques, can appear anywhere on the body but are most commonly found on the elbows, knees, scalp, and lower back. Psoriasis occurs when the immune system mistakenly triggers inflammation, causing skin cells to grow too quickly. The exact cause is unknown, but it is believed to be influenced by genetic and environmental factors. Psoriasis is a lifelong condition with periods of flare-ups and remission.

Brand Name	Generic Name	Classification
DHS Tar Shampoo, Tegrin, Zetar	Coal Tar	Kertoplastic
Fluticasone, Budesonide	Corticosteroids	Steroids

Other 1st line treatment include Vitamin D Analogs and Topical Retinoids but they will likely not be on your exam thus they are not highlighted

Main System Use

Coal Tar :
keratoplastic agent, which means it influences the growth and regeneration of the outer layer of the skin, known as the stratum corneum; helps normalize the growth of excessive skin by reducing the rapid division and growth of skin cells.

Corticosteroids :
Inhibiting the production of inflammatory cytokines, including interleukins and tumor necrosis factor (TNF)

Pearls

Coal Tar :

- Avoid open wounds/may cause skin irritation
- Protect from sunlight and UV light

Corticosteroids :

- Monitor glucose control
- Monitor bone health
- Possible increase risk for infections
- Taper appropriately
- Can increase intraocular pressure
- Pt with hx of mood disorder monitor

DERMATOLOGY

Acne Rosacea

Definition of the disease

Acne Rosacea, commonly known as rosacea, is a chronic inflammatory skin condition that primarily affects the face. It is characterized by persistent redness, visible blood vessels, and small, red, pus-filled bumps resembling acne. Rosacea most commonly affects the central part of the face, including the cheeks, nose, forehead, and chin. The exact cause is unknown, but it is thought to be a combination of genetic predisposition, abnormal immune response, and environmental triggers such as sun exposure, spicy foods, alcohol, and stress. Rosacea can worsen over time if untreated, leading to thickened skin, particularly on the nose (rhinophyma), or eye involvement (ocular rosacea). Treatment typically involves topical or oral medications, lifestyle modifications, and in some cases, laser therapy to control symptoms and manage flare-ups.

Brand Name	Generic Name	Classification
Topical Flagyl/ Metrogel	Metronidazole	Antifungal
Ery-tab, Eryc EryPed, Illotycin	Erythromycin	Macrolide
Cleocin, Clindagel, Dalacin	Clindamycin	Lincosamide
Finacea	Azelic Acid	Dicarboxylic

Acne Rosacea

Main System Use

Clindamycin : It works by binding to the 50S ribosomal subunit of bacterial ribosomes, which are essential for protein production in bacterial cells. This interference with protein synthesis disrupts bacterial growth and replication.

Erythromycin : Involving its ability to inhibit bacterial protein synthesis

Metronidazole : Disruption of DNA synthesis in certain microorganisms, leading to the inhibition of their growth and replication

Azelic Acid : Inhibit the growth of Propionibacterium acnes, a type of bacteria that plays a role in the development of acne and also promotes skin cell turnover and normalizes shedding dead skin

Pearls

Clindamycin :

- Check for cross allergies
- Monitor for GI upset
- Increased risk of Cdiff
- Avoid Alcohol
- No: hx of pseudomembranous colitis
- Renal and Hepatic monitoring

Avoid alcohol :

- Avoid in 1st trimester
- Monitor liver function
- GI upset(metallic, n/v, diarrhea)
- Headache/dizziness/dry mouth
- Can increase yeast infections
- Monitor for leukopenia and thrombocytopenia

Erythromycin :

- SE: Nausea/Diarrhea/Skin
- Reactions
- Increase Risk of Cdiff
- Avoid Alcohol
- Renal and Hepatic function monitoring
- No: Cardiac Arrhythmias/ Long QT Syndrome

DERMATOLOGY

Tinea Corporis

Definition of the disease

Tinea Corporis, also known as ringworm of the body, is a superficial fungal infection affecting the skin. It is caused by dermatophyte fungi, typically from the Trichophyton or Microsporum species. The infection presents as red, circular, scaly patches with clear or less inflamed centers, often forming a "ring-like" appearance. These lesions can appear on various parts of the body, excluding the scalp, groin, and feet, and may cause itching, discomfort, and sometimes a slight burning sensation. Tinea corporis is spread through direct contact with infected individuals, animals, or contaminated objects such as towels or clothing.

Brand Name	Generic Name	Classification
Lotrimin/ Nizoral/ Monistat	Miconazole/ Clotrimazole/ Ketoconazol	Antifungal

Main System Use

Antifungal :
By targeting the fungal cells and disrupting their structure or function inhibiting the synthesis of ergosterol, leading to cell membrane disruption

Pearls

- Avoid open wounds/may cause skin irritation
- Protect from sunlight and UV light
- Infection Control

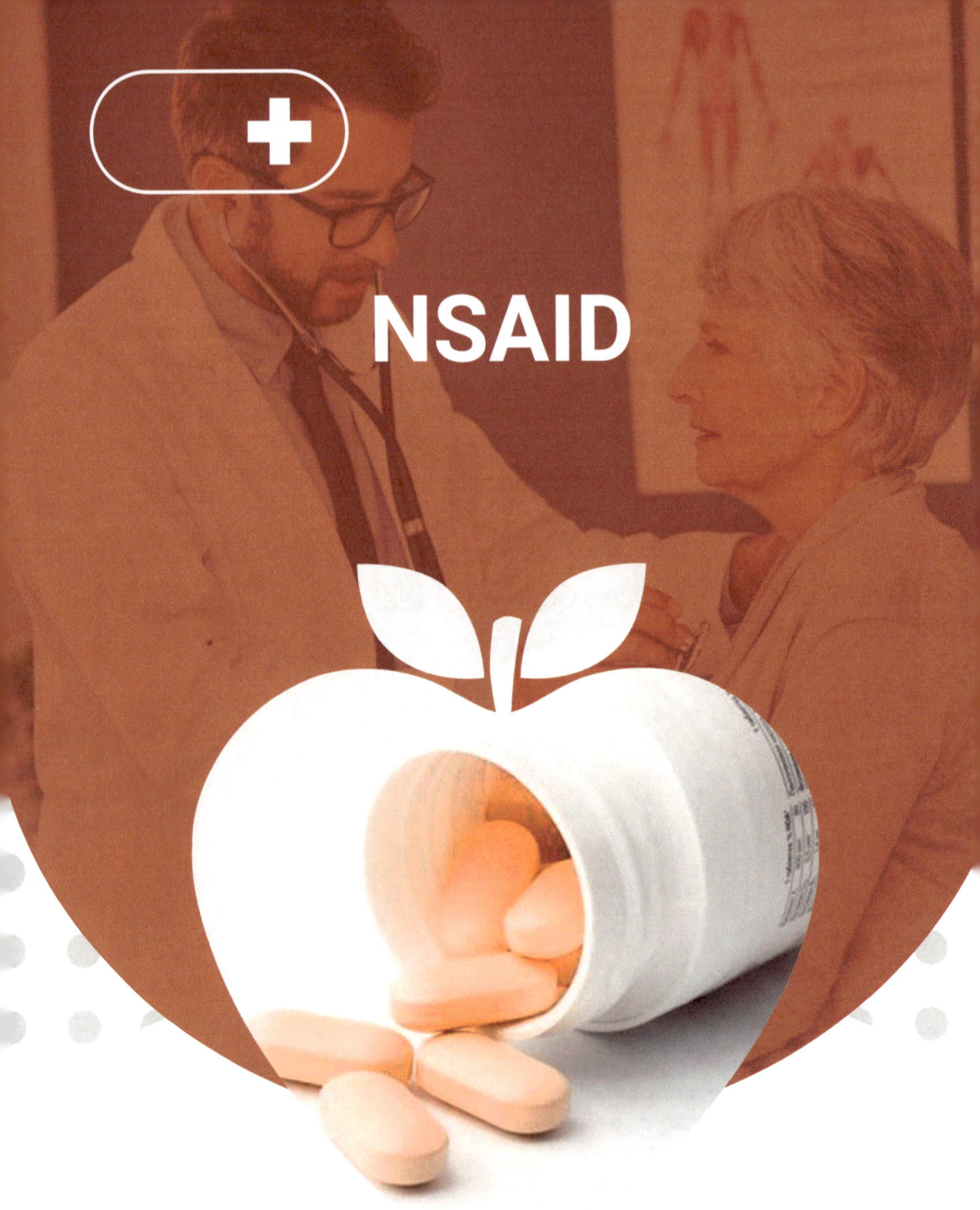

NSAID

Latrina Walden™
Exam Solutions

NSAID

Definition of the disease

NSAID (Non-Steroidal Anti-Inflammatory Drug) is a class of medications used to relieve pain, reduce inflammation, and lower fever. Unlike corticosteroids, NSAIDs do not contain steroids but work by inhibiting the enzymes cyclooxygenase-1 (COX-1) and cyclooxygenase-2 (COX-2), which play a key role in the production of prostaglandins—chemicals in the body that mediate inflammation and pain. Common examples of NSAIDs include ibuprofen, aspirin, naproxen, and ketoprofen. They are commonly used to treat conditions such as arthritis, menstrual cramps, muscle pain, and headaches. While effective for pain relief and inflammation, NSAIDs can have side effects, including gastrointestinal irritation, increased risk of bleeding, and potential kidney damage with long-term use.

Brand Name	Generic Name	Classification
Aleve	Naproxen	NSAIDS
Celebrex	Celecoxib	NSAIDS
Advil/ Motrin	Clindamycin	NSAIDS
Voltaren	Diclofenac	NSAIDS
Mobic	Meloxicam	NSAIDS

***1st line treatment for Tension Headaches*
***1st line treatment for Gout*
***1st line treatment for Rheumatoid Arthritis*

NSAID

Main System Use

Inhibiting the activity of cyclooxygenase enzymes, particularly COX-1 and COX-2. These enzymes play a crucial role in the production of prostaglandins, which are lipid compounds that promote inflammation, pain, and fever. COX-1 is constitutively present in various tissues and is involved in normal physiological functions, while COX-2 is induced during inflammation.

Pearls

- Caution GI irritation/bleeding/ulcers
- Caution those w/ Heart disease
- Monitor Renal function
- Consider PPI
- Contraindications for those antiplatelet drugs
- Caution asthma/bronchospasms

PSYCHIATRIC

Analgesic / Antipyretic

Definition of the disease

Non-Opioid Analgesics are a class of medications used to relieve pain without containing opioids. They work by either reducing inflammation or blocking pain signals in the body. Common examples include acetaminophen, such as Tylenol, which is effective for reducing pain and fever but does not have significant anti-inflammatory effects, and non-steroidal anti-inflammatory drugs (NSAIDs), such as ibuprofen and naproxen, which help reduce pain, inflammation, and fever. These medications are typically used for mild to moderate pain and are preferred for their lower risk of addiction compared to opioids.

Brand Name	Generic Name	Classification
Paracetamol/ Tylenol	Acetaminophen	Analgesic/ Antipyretic

Main System Use

Reduce the production of prostaglandins in the brain acting in the central nervous system

Pearls

- **Do not exceed 4g per day**
- Overdose leads to Hepatoxicity
- May increase bleeding with warfarin therapy
- May alter blood glucose monitoring
- Monitor Renal function <Alcohol can increase>

NOTES

NOTES

ISBN 978-1-7369010-6-9

9 781736 901069

Made in the USA
Las Vegas, NV
03 November 2026

57424597R00046